TRUSTING GOD FOR RENEWED LIFE

C·R·E·A·T·I·O·N Health

LIFE GUIDE #5

For Individual Study and Small Group Use

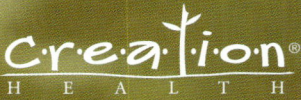

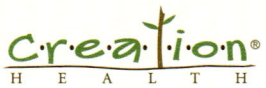

CREATION Health Life Guide #5
Copyright © MMXII by Florida Hospital
Published by Florida Hospital Publishing
900 Winderley Place, Suite 1600
Maitland, Florida 32751

To Extend the Health and Healing Ministry of Christ

Publisher and Editor-in-Chief:	Todd Chobotar
Managing Editor:	David Biebel, DMin
Production:	Lillian Boyd
Promotion:	Laurel Prizigley
Copy Editor:	Pamela Nordberg
Author Photography:	Timothy Brown
Design:	Carter Design, Inc.
Peer Reviewers:	Amaryllis Sanchez-Wohlever, MD; Robert Hayes Bradford Eakins, MDiv; Barbara Olsen, MACL Karen Tilstra, PhD; Sabine Vatel, DMin Andy McDonald, DMin; Tim Goff, MDiv Rick Szilagyi, DMin; Gerald Wasmer, MDiv Andre VanHeerden; Paul Campoli, MDiv

Publisher's Note: This book is not intended to replace a one-on-one relationship with a qualified healthcare professional, but as a sharing of knowledge and information from the research and experience of the author. You are advised and encouraged to consult with your healthcare professional in all matters relating to your health and the health of your family. The publisher and author disclaim any liability arising directly or indirectly from the use of this book.

The author assumes full responsibility for the accuracy of all facts and quotations as cited in this book. CREATION Health is a registered trademark of Florida Hospital. All rights reserved.

NOT TO BE REPRODUCED
No portion of this book may be reproduced, stored in a retrieval system, or transmitted in any form or by any means – electronic, mechanical, photocopy, recording, or any other – except for brief quotations in printed reviews, without the prior written permission of the publisher. All rights reserved.

Unless otherwise indicated, all Scripture quotations are taken from the Holy Bible, New Living Translation, copyright © 1996, 2004 by Tyndale House Publishers, Inc., Wheaton, Illinois 60189. All other Scripture references are from the following sources: The Holy Bible, New International Version (NIV), copyright © 1973, 1978, 1984 by Biblica, Inc. Used by permission of Zondervan. The Holy Bible, Revised Standard Version (RSV), copyright © 1946, 1952, 1971 by the National Council of the Churches of Christ. The Holy Bible, King James Version (KJV). The Holy Bible, New King James Version (NKJV), copyright © 1982 by Thomas Nelson, Inc. The Message (MSG), copyright © by Eugene H. Peterson 1993, 1994, 1995, 1996, 2000, 2001, 2002. Used by permission of NAVPress Publishing Group. Good News Translation ® (Today's English Version, Second Edition) Copyright © 1992 American Bible Society. All Scriptures used by permission. All rights reserved.

For volume discounts please contact special sales at:
HealthProducts@FLHosp.org | 407-303-1929

Printed in the United States of America.
PR 14 13 12 11 10 9 8 7 6 5 4 3 2 1
ISBN: 978-0-9887406-4-8

For more life-changing resources visit:
**FloridaHospitalPublishing.com
Healthy100Churches.org
CREATIONHealth.com
Healthy100.org**

CONTENTS

Introduction — Welcome to CREATION Health — 4

1. God's Search for Trust — 6
2. A Savior We Can Trust — 18
3. Understanding Trust — 30
4. Trusting God for New Life — 42
5. Benefits of Trust — 54
6. Trusting God's Word — 66
7. Building Trust Through Scripture — 76
8. Building Trust Through Prayer — 88

About the Author — 101

Notes — 102

Resources — 105

DOWNLOAD YOUR FREE LEADER RESOURCE

Are you a small group leader? We've created a special resource to help you lead an effective CREATION Health discussion group. Download at: **CREATIONHealth.com/LeaderResources**

WELCOME TO CREATION HEALTH

Congratulations on your choice to use this resource to improve your life! Whether you are new to the concept of CREATION Health or are a seasoned expert, this book was created for you. CREATION Health is a faith-based health and wellness program based on the Bible's Creation story. This book is part of a Life Guide series seeking to help you apply eight elegantly simple principles for living life to the full.

The letters of the CREATION acronym stand for:

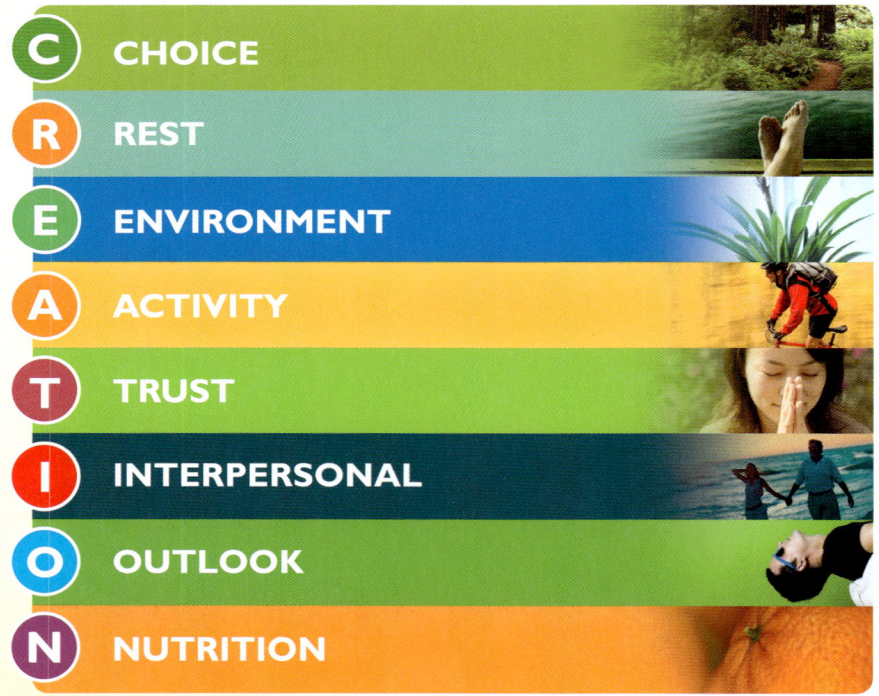

- **C** CHOICE
- **R** REST
- **E** ENVIRONMENT
- **A** ACTIVITY
- **T** TRUST
- **I** INTERPERSONAL
- **O** OUTLOOK
- **N** NUTRITION

In John 10:10 Jesus said, "I have come that they may have life, and have it to the full" (NIV). The Greek word used for life is "zoe," which means the absolute fullness of life…genuine life…a life that is active, satisfying, and filled with joy.

That is why CREATION Health takes a life-transforming approach to total person wellness – mentally, physically, spiritually, and socially – with the eight universal principles of health. Where did these principles come from?

The book of Genesis describes how God created the earth and made a special garden called Eden as a home for his first two children, Adam and Eve. One of the first and finest gifts given to them was abundant health. By examining the Creation story we can learn much about feeling fit and living long, fulfilling lives today.

As you begin this journey toward an improved lifestyle, remember that full health is more than the absence of disease and its symptoms. It's a realization that God desires each of his children – people like you and me whom he loves and cares about – to have the best that this life can offer. It is trusting that your Creator has a plan for your life.

Is there any good parent who doesn't want the best for their child? No. So it makes sense that God would want his best for us. Naturally, human freedom of choice sometimes makes life messy, so not everything can or will be perfect as it once was. But that doesn't mean we shouldn't take a good look at the earliest records of humans found in the Bible to see if there is something special that can be gleaned.

This book – and the other seven in the Life Guide series – takes a deep dive into CREATION Health and translates the fundamental concepts into easy-to-follow steps. These guides include many questions designed to help you or your small group plumb the depths of every principle and learn strategies for integrating the things you learn into everyday life. As a result, you will discover that embracing the CREATION Health prescription can help restore health, happiness, balance, and joy to life.

The CREATION Health Lifestyle has a long, proven history of wellness and longevity – worldwide! People just like you are making a few simple changes in their lives and living longer, fuller lives. They are getting healthy, staying healthy, and are able to do the things they love, well into their later years. Now is the time to join them by transforming your habits into a healthy lifestyle.

If you would like to learn more about the many resources available, visit **CREATIONHealth.com**. If you would like to learn more about how to live to a Healthy 100, visit **Healthy100.org** or visit **Healthy100Churches.org**.

Welcome to CREATION Health,

Todd Chobotar
Publisher and Editor-in-Chief

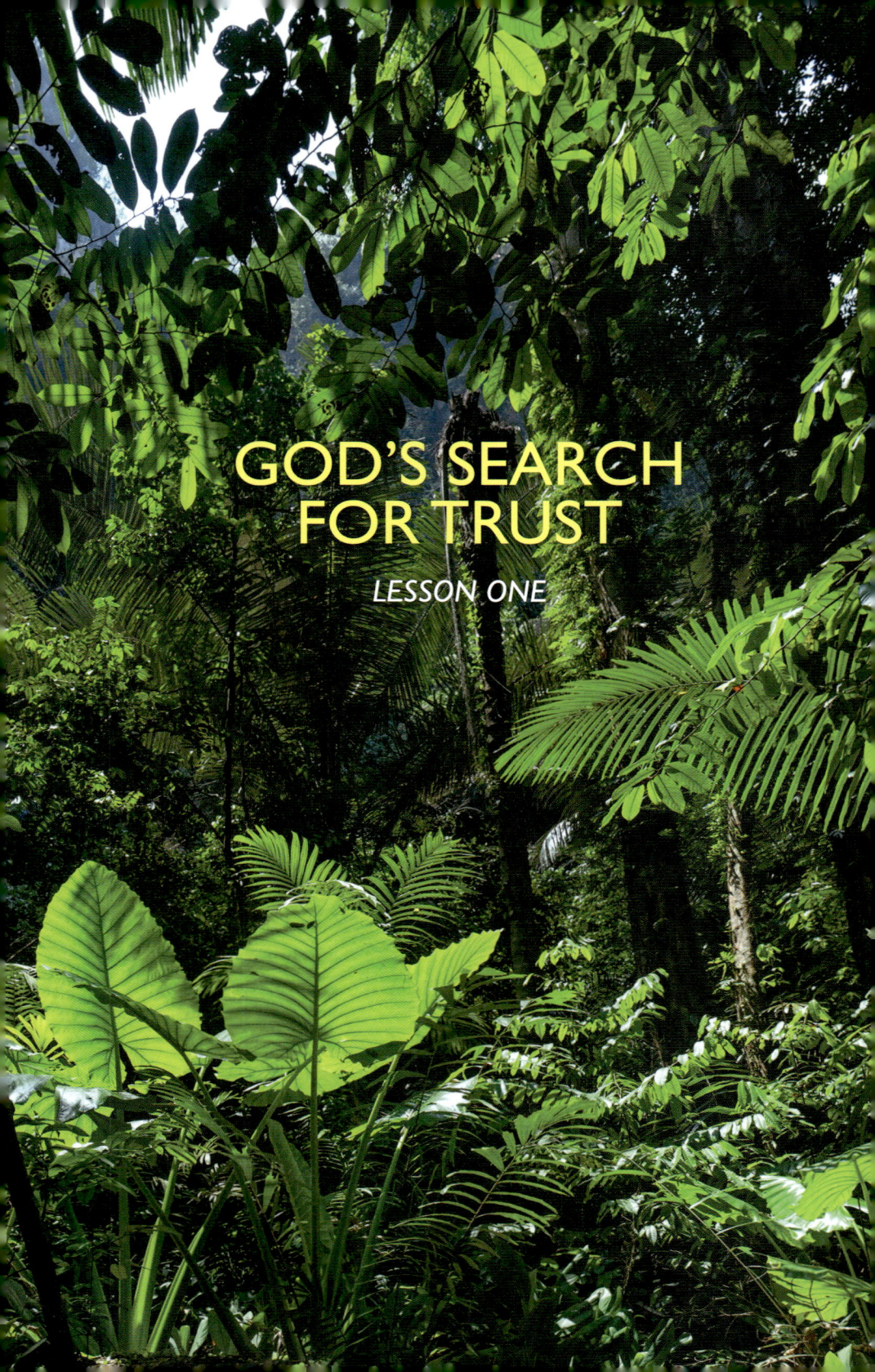

GOD'S SEARCH FOR TRUST

LESSON ONE

WARM UP

Choose one or both questions to discuss (if in a group setting) or write out your answers on a separate sheet (for individual use):

1. **Describe a favorite thing you think about during quiet times.**[1]

....
....
....
....
....
....
....

2. **What is your most effective means of relieving stress?**[2]

....
....
....
....
....
....
....

> "The only One who can truly satisfy the human heart is the One who made it."
> **MARCHIA MILLER**

DISCOVERY

This lesson provides a brief overview of God's intense efforts to enter into a trust relationship with the inhabitants of planet Earth. The storyline is based on Scripture with some small parts of the narrative filled in through the use of imagination.

Before our world was brought into existence, millions of angels were already joyfully carrying out important assignments in God's far-flung kingdom. There never seemed to be enough beings, however, to satisfy God's compassion. In spite of the vast size of the creation he already cared for, he craved more opportunities to give of himself to others.

As a result of this yearning to love, God decided to establish planet Earth in a non-descript area of the cosmos and populate it with humans. He could envision it in breathtaking detail. As he shared his plans, the angels thrilled at the prospect. They had seen before what God's immense imagination and power could produce. They knew from experience that his proposal would outstrip anything their own ingenuity might envision.

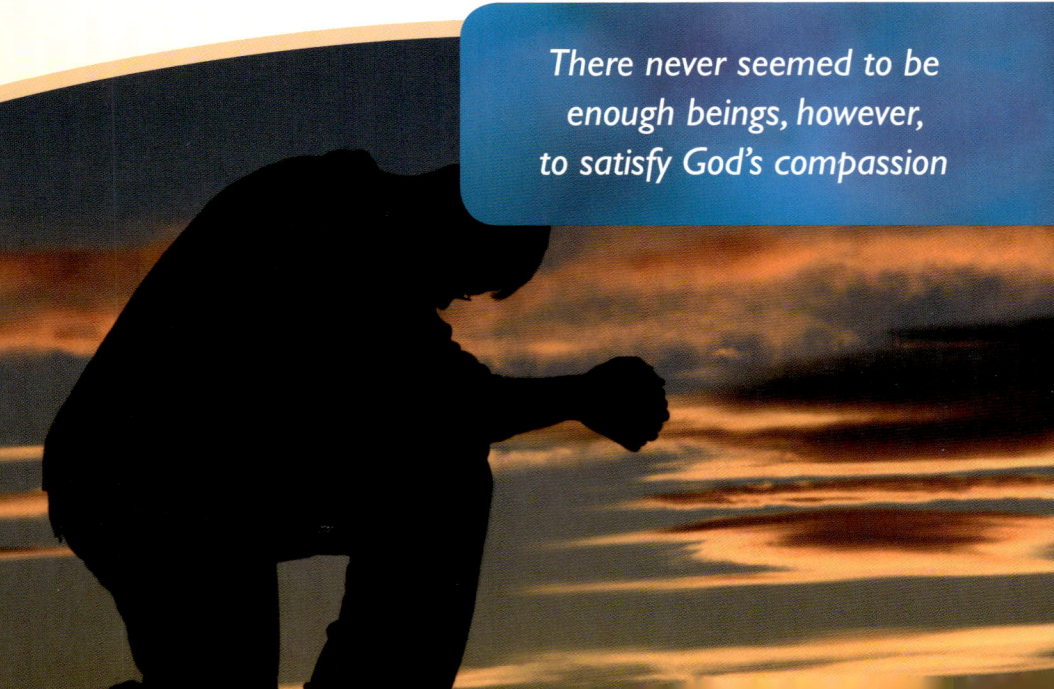

There never seemed to be enough beings, however, to satisfy God's compassion

The book of Genesis reveals how God's exquisite dream became reality (see Gen. 1 and 2). Over the course of a few days, God's word transformed our globe from a desolate void into a teeming landscape and verdant sea. Barren fields suddenly abounded with multi-colored, fragrant flowers. Majestic trees arched skyward. Animals of all shapes and sizes roamed the lush hills and valleys. A cornucopia of birds, from chickadees to eagles, populated the skies. Fish and warm-blooded creatures glided, squirmed, leaped, and darted in the liquid produced by the life-giving chemical reaction between two parts hydrogen and one part oxygen.

All was now prepared for the arrival of the crowning achievement of God's intentions. According to the book of Genesis, God created the first man, Adam, by personally shaping him from clay like a master sculptor (Gen. 2:7). The artistry and complexity of it all were staggering – the regal head, multi-billion celled brain, interconnected bodily systems, and countless interacting elements.

The infinite God then paused, stared deeply into the young man's lifeless, hand-crafted eyes, and breathed life into his mighty frame. The earthly gray of the muddy clay instantly gave way to the pink of blood-infused organs and skin. Adam drew in several deep draughts of air. His eyes blinked and his fingers flexed. Within moments he stood, looked directly at his Creator, then instinctively knelt in adoration.

Soon thereafter, God created Eve with exquisite gentleness and care. She was breathtakingly beautiful, full of talent, intelligence, and myriad capabilities.

The husband and wife team spent the rest of their first day in animated conversation with their maker. They thanked him profusely for the marvelous garden home and other gifts he had so generously provided.

For an unspecified amount of time, months or years we do not know, Adam and Eve enjoyed regular, face-to-face, personal time with the One who is larger than galaxies, who is unfettered by time and space, who is the source of all life, and has existed from eternity past. The all-powerful, all-knowing, all-present God poured himself into the first couple as parent, guide, and friend.

The three of them laughed together, sang together, walked, and dreamed together. God was delighted to explain the intricacies of the natural world he had manufactured, covering subjects as diverse as design, physics, biology, chemistry, physiology, landscaping, and horticulture. Adam and Eve's innate genius eagerly absorbed it all. *They learned to trust God completely because they knew him to be utterly trustworthy.* The communication was clear, open, honest, undistorted.

The Creator gave Adam and Eve free rein, unlimited opportunities, and enormous privileges. Just one restriction. He told them, "You are free to eat from any tree in the garden; but you must not eat from the tree of the knowledge of good and evil" (Gen. 2:16–17, NIV). *It was a small request, designed to deepen trust.* It provided them with an essential opportunity to exercise freedom of choice, which is at the heart of any genuine trust relationship.

Offering such a choice, however, also came with the inherent danger of choosing wrongly, of rebelling, of not trusting. By any reasonable calculation, that downside should have been a remote possibility, a miniscule likelihood, considering all of the stupendous positives that would flow from choosing well. God carefully explained the gift of free will and its potential for great good or devastating ill. "You can always trust my love," he assured repeatedly.

The devil now entered the story and used a clever ruse to capture Eve's attention. He began speaking to her through a cunning reptile. Eve was intrigued. Like any charlatan, the evil one initially spent time winning her confidence and surreptitiously getting her to let down her guard.

Their sociable discussion then took an ominous turn. The serpent raised the issue of God's one restriction and urged her to eat what God had specifically instructed the couple to avoid. "God isn't being truthful," he advised. "He's holding back knowledge that you should have" (see Gen. 3:4–5). Inextricably, horribly, instead of trusting her maker and friend, she chose badly and partook from the tree. Adam soon assessed what had happened and chose to rebel as well.

Quickly everything changed. Adam and Eve's mutual decision had inevitable moral and natural consequences. It would be like us deliberately putting sand in the gas tank of our car. The principle of cause and effect played out in a cascade of terrible transformations. An uncommon chill seeped into the air. A feeling of dread displaced any previous joy.

Heartbroken, God could instantly envision the painful future and was grieved to the core. Only the Creator could fully understand the awful outcomes that would inexorably ensue. The heart of infinite love suffered infinite hurt. His songs dried up and tears flowed freely.

Rather than responding to Adam and Eve with anger, God reached out to them with infinite compassion. In the face of rejection, his only thought was to draw near and be with them as he had done so many times before.

> The all-powerful, all-knowing, all-present God poured himself into the first couple as parent, guide, and friend.

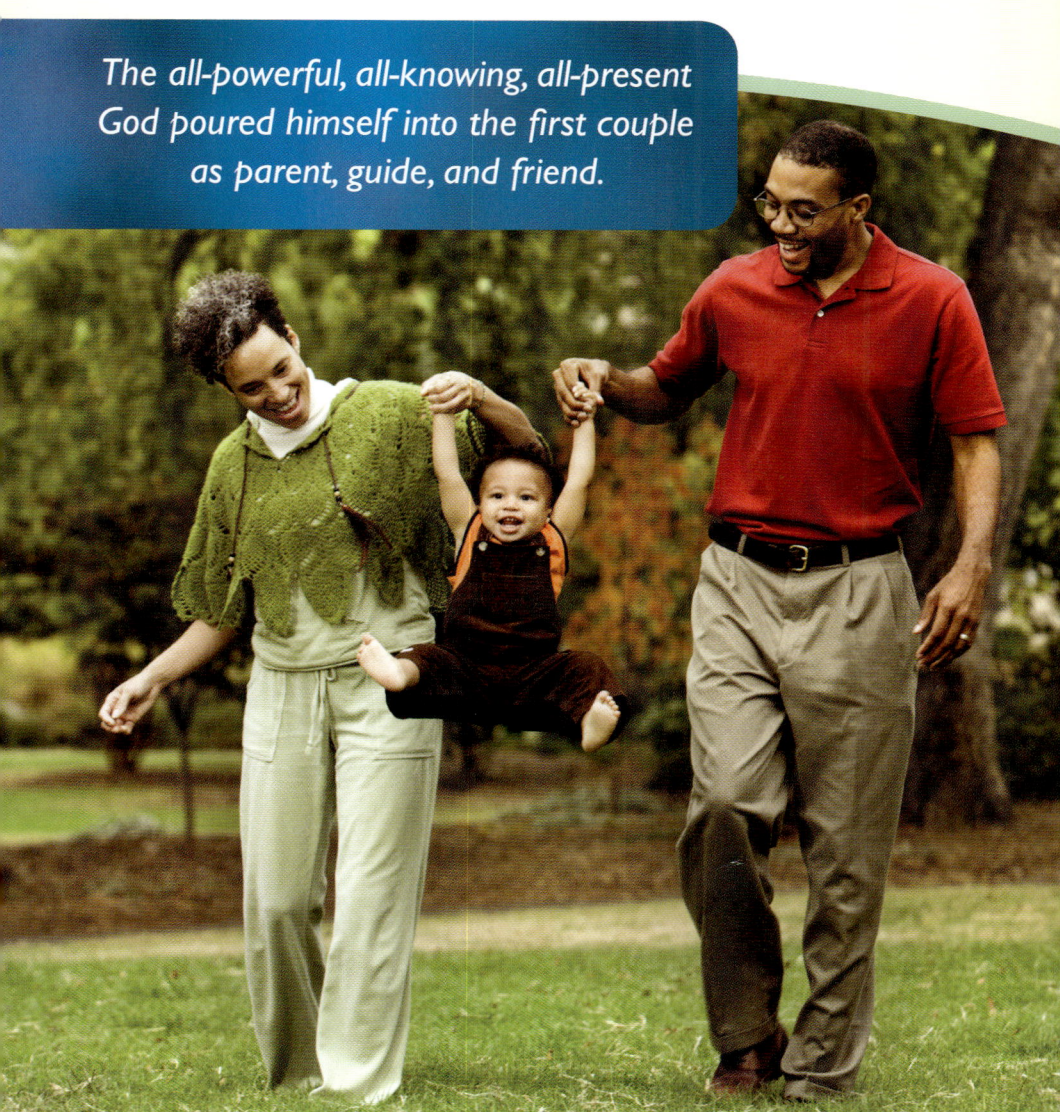

The first couple sensed his presence and hid in shame. God then called out with voice-cracking emotion, "Where are you?" (Gen. 3:9, NIV). They soon emerged and told him they were "afraid" (Gen. 3:10). How that dreadful word must have slammed into God's heart! The mutual trust he had so carefully cultivated now lay in ruins. The relationship between Adam and Eve itself suffered as well. Intimacy and selflessness quickly morphed into suspicion and blame as they accused each other and even God himself.

As a result of Adam and Eve's decision, all subsequent human relationships became infected with the cancer of distrust. Like a mutant gene, it passed from one generation to the next. Tension and misunderstanding grew. As the human family expanded, selfishness became the norm, creating untold fractures and separations (see Gen. 4–6).

The God of love found himself increasingly marginalized by subsequent generations. People came to label him as judgmental, uncaring, and manipulative. Many relegated him to a minor, distant role. Others began doubting his very existence.

In the face of such appalling rejection and mischaracterization, God's only desire was to help his wayward offspring. Over the centuries, God has tried in every imaginable way to convince his earthly children that he loves them unconditionally and can indeed be trusted. From that perspective, the Bible is the greatest love story of all time.

In order to counteract humanity's pervasive misconceptions, God raised up champions of faith to serve as messengers and role models. Noah spent decades building a massive ark based solely on his confidence in God's words of warning. Abraham left the security of his extensive lands and possessions because he trusted God's call to pull up stakes and move without clear direction (see Hebrews 11).

Joseph's faith in God remained firm even after being sold into slavery by his brothers and spending years in unjust imprisonment. Looking back on those experiences years later as a great leader in Egypt, Joseph could affirm to his siblings, "Don't you see, you planned evil against me, but God used those same plans for my good" (Gen. 50:20, MSG).

Many other names could be added. Job, for instance, endured horrendous loss but nonetheless testified that he would still trust God no matter what the future held (Job 13:14–16).

In addition to the witness of individuals, God also chose to raise up an entire nation of people who would hopefully testify collectively to the world regarding his true character and intentions. He delivered the Israelites from Egyptian slavery in spectacular fashion and gave them amazing opportunities to know him intimately and relate to him in love.

God spoke words of great affection and optimism regarding Israel, such as when he told them:

> *I have loved you, my people, with an everlasting love.*
> *With unfailing love I have drawn you to myself (Jer. 31:3).*

> *Since you were precious in My sight,*
> *You have been honored,*
> *And I have loved you (Isa. 43:4, NKJV).*

> *For I know the thoughts that I think toward you, says the Lord, thoughts of peace and not of evil, to give you a future and a hope (Jer. 29:11, NKJV).*

> *In order to counteract humanity's pervasive misconceptions, God raised up champions of faith to serve as messengers and role models.*

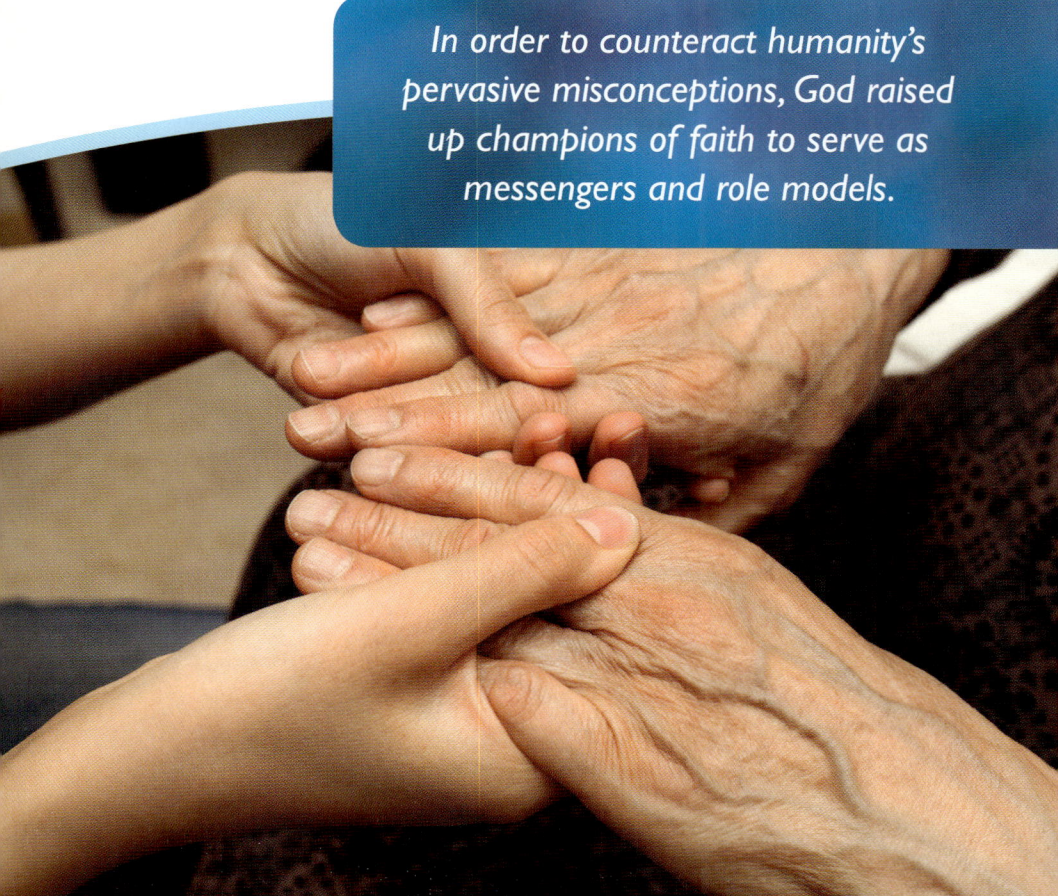

The nation did, in fact, experience periods of success and faithfulness. But all too often they rebelled and were defeated. During these heartbreaking times, God uttered words of grief and loss, as in the book of Hosea:

> *When Israel was a child, I loved him*
> *and called him out of Egypt as my son.*
> *But the more I called to him,*
> *the more he turned away from me . . .*
> *Yet I was the one who taught Israel to walk.*
> *I took my people up in my arms,*
> *but they did not acknowledge that I took care of them.*
> *I drew them to me with affection and love.*
> *I picked them up and held them to my cheek;*
> *I bent down to them and fed them.*
> *[But] they refuse to return to me . . .*
> *They insist on turning away from me (Hosea 11:1–7, GNT).*

Despite the waywardness of the multitudes, there were individuals within the nation of Israel whose dedication and commitment stood out far above the rest. Their leader, Moses, trusted God's assurances enough to risk his life confronting Pharaoh. He also exhibited extraordinary confidence in God during his forty terribly challenging years as CEO.

When Israel was taken captive by the heathen nation of Babylon, the faithfulness of three young Jewish men, Shadrach, Meshach, and Abednego, provided a spine-tingling endorsement of God's character. After refusing to bow down to King Nebuchadnezzar's statue, the three were thrown into a super-heated furnace. Their miraculous deliverance caused the king to issue the following amazing decree to all of his leaders: "Praise be to the God of Shadrach, Meshach and Abednego, who has sent his angel and rescued his servants! *They trusted in him* and defied the king's command and were willing to give up their lives rather than serve or worship any god except their own God" (Daniel 3:28, NIV, emphasis added).

The prophet Daniel, who also endured captivity in Babylon, underscored God's trustworthiness when he chose loyalty to him even though it meant being thrown into a den of ravenous lions.

Tragically, despite these powerful exceptions, Old Testament Israel ultimately turned away from God's plan, and he had to look elsewhere.

Two thousand years ago, God established a new beginning by sending his own son, Jesus Christ, into this world as a helpless babe. God would now reach humans by becoming human. Hurting people could look directly into his compassionate eyes and hear his words of hope and healing. The savior came specifically to give us the fullest possible revelation of God's limitless love. He explained clearly, "He who has seen Me has seen the Father" (John 14:9, NKJV).

Through both word and deed, Christ established for all time the truth about God and his trustworthiness. Jesus dedicated his life to developing transformative love relationships with hurting, suffering humanity and overcoming the devil's falsehoods and distortions. Many responded positively, but others took offense, spurned his love, and nailed him to a cross.

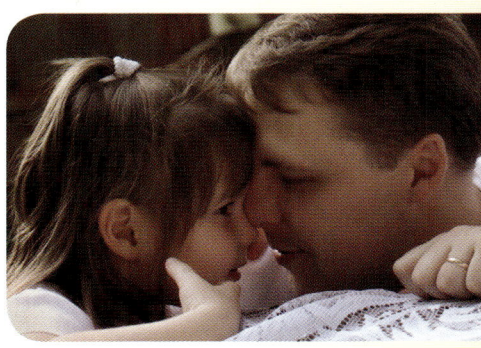

The New Testament church then emerged after Jesus' death and resurrection to carry on the work he had so wonderfully established. Paul, Peter, John, James, and other early Christian leaders launched a movement that impacted the world.

The epic story of God's search for relationships of trust continues to be played out in our own day. Such a relationship can provide us with wonderful new dimensions of wholeness and fulfillment now and open the way to someday spending all eternity with the One who loves us so.

As we consider our own understanding of God, the encouraging testimony of the psalmist David echoes down through time, providing a window into the heart of the loving redeemer he knew so well:

> *Blessed be the Lord,*
> *Because He has heard the voice of my supplications!*
> *The Lord is my strength and my shield;*
> *My heart trusted in Him, and I am helped;*
> *Therefore my heart greatly rejoices,*
> *And with my song I will praise Him (Psalm 28:6–8, NKJV).*
>
> *Oh, taste and see that the Lord is good;*
> *Blessed is the man who trusts in Him! (Psalm 34:8, NKJV).*

DISCUSSION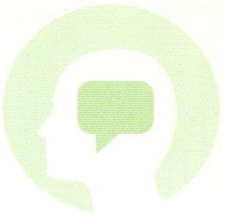

What does this overview say to you about God?

Describe one of your favorite examples in Scripture of trusting God.

What are some common misconceptions people have about God today?

What is it about sin that fractures relationships?

Describe a modern-day experience that might help you feel some of God's sense of loss and sadness when Adam and Eve sinned.

What are some of the differences between serving God out of love and serving him out of fear?

What are some ways we can hide from God?

How can we learn to trust God more fully?

SHARING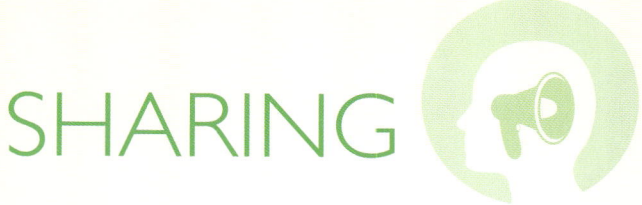

OPPORTUNITY #1

If studying in a group, this section is about an opportunity for you to be a blessing to someone outside of your small group and to also deepen the impact of the lesson on your own life. The group is encouraged to discuss at the end of each meeting what aspects of the lesson they might like to share with someone at home, work, or in the community if the opportunity arises. An "Abundant Living Thought" at the end of each lesson is one possibility of something to pass along.

Start each day asking God to provide opportunities to share, and then keep your radar up.

You can be an ambassador and reach people with the good news that abundant living is available to all.

ABUNDANT LIVING THOUGHT

Over the centuries, God has tried in every imaginable way to convince his earthly children that he can indeed be trusted.

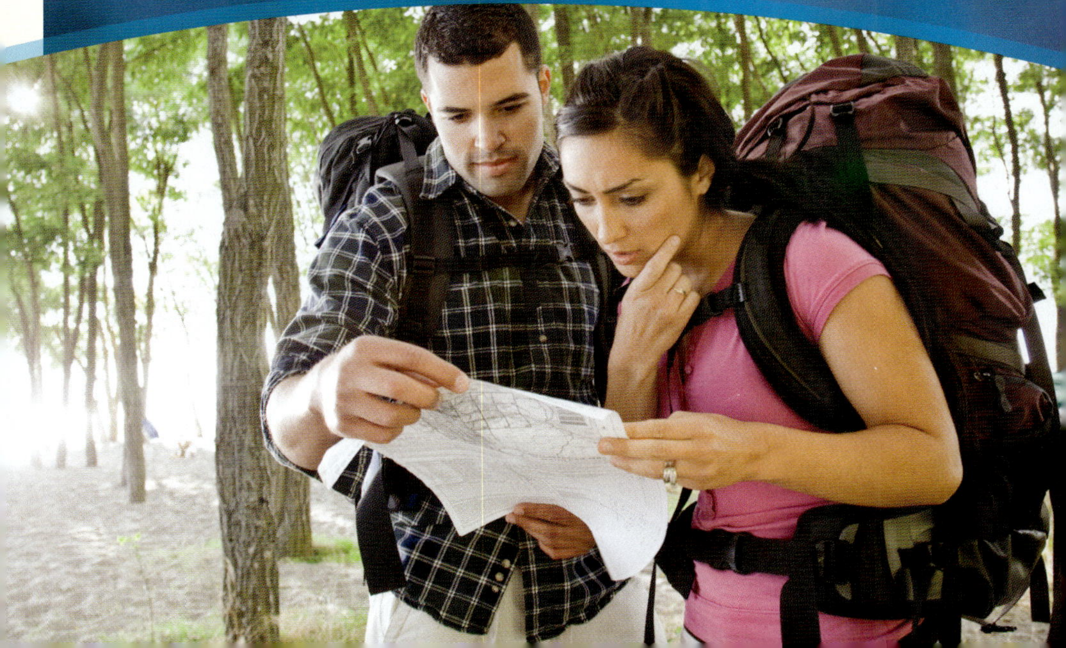

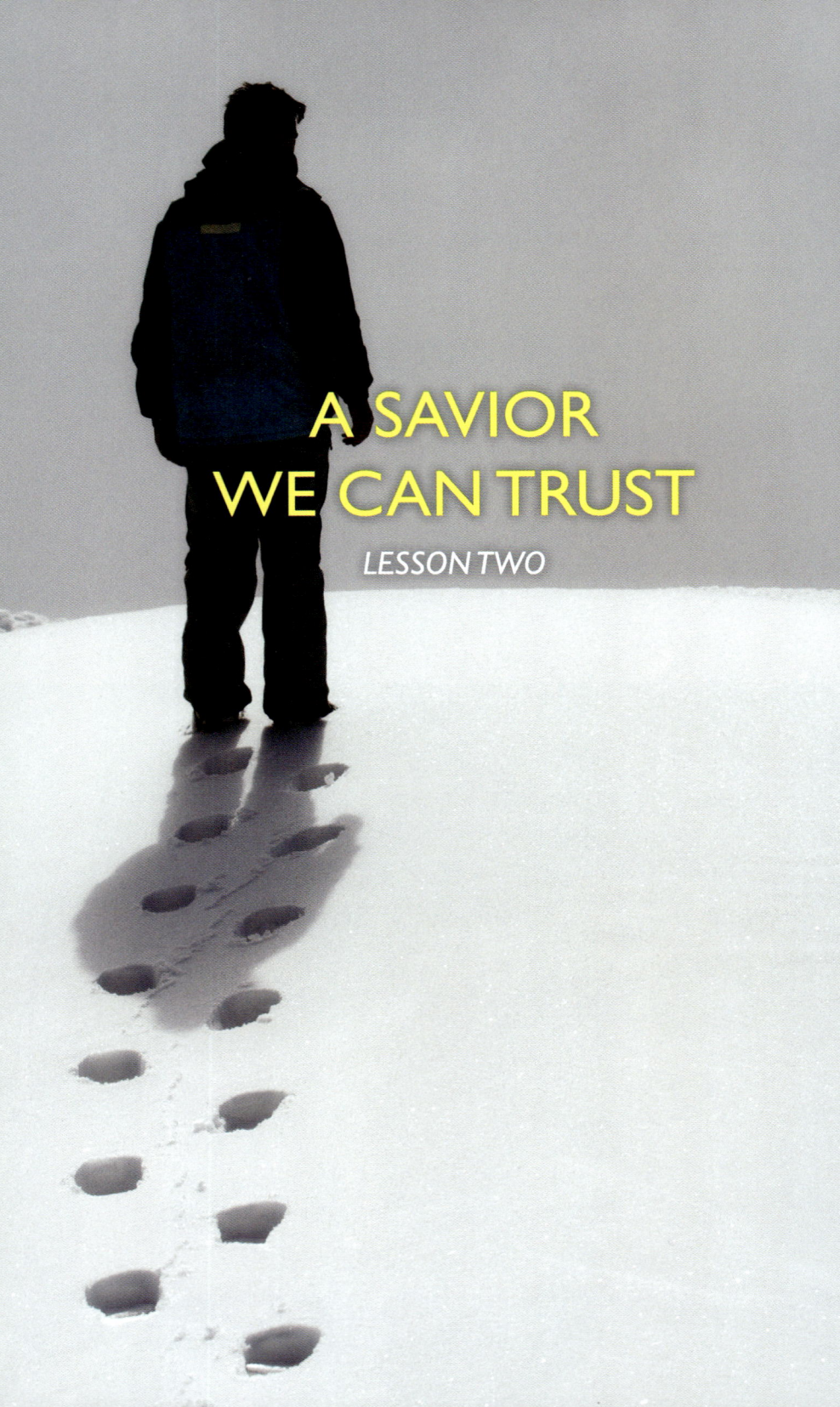

WARM UP

Feedback: In what ways did God open the door last week for you to share some part of the lesson with someone else?

....
....
....
....

Choose one or both questions to discuss (if in a group setting), or write out your answers on a separate sheet (for individual use):

1. **Describe one of your proudest moments in life.**[3]

....
....
....

2. **Briefly share something interesting you were told about one of your ancestors.**[4]

....
....
....

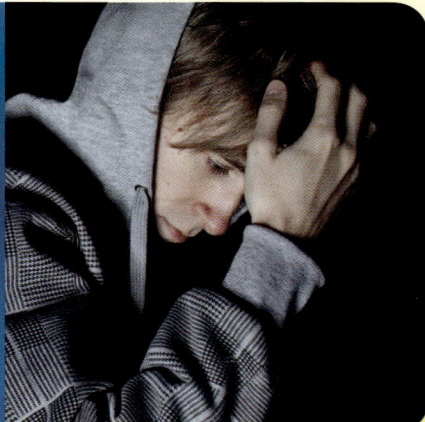

Sometimes we simply cannot understand, but is it enough to know who does?

DR. DAVID BIEBEL

DISCOVERY

My wife and I used to live in very rural Pownal, Maine. Downtown consisted of a convenience store, an auto repair shop, and the town hall. When it came time to update the registration on your car, you went to the home of Mrs. Hooper, the town clerk.

In stark contrast to Pownal's under-the-radar profile was a world-class department store only ten miles away that specialized in outdoor equipment and clothing. They had a stellar, national reputation for being trustworthy, not only because of the high quality of their goods, but especially as a result of their amazing return policy. You could return anything at any time for any reason. No questions asked.

Somewhat skeptical, I decided to test the policy and brought in a pair of their boots I had purchased six years before. In my opinion, the tread had worn more than expected. I approached the return counter sheepishly and placed the boots on top. The clerk smiled warmly, grabbed the boots, put them on the floor behind her, and asked kindly, "Would you like cash or a new pair?" I paused to retrieve my chin from the floor and stammered, "Cash, please." They get taken advantage of periodically, but their reputation for having the most generous, trusted return policy on the planet has built an exceptionally loyal base of customers.

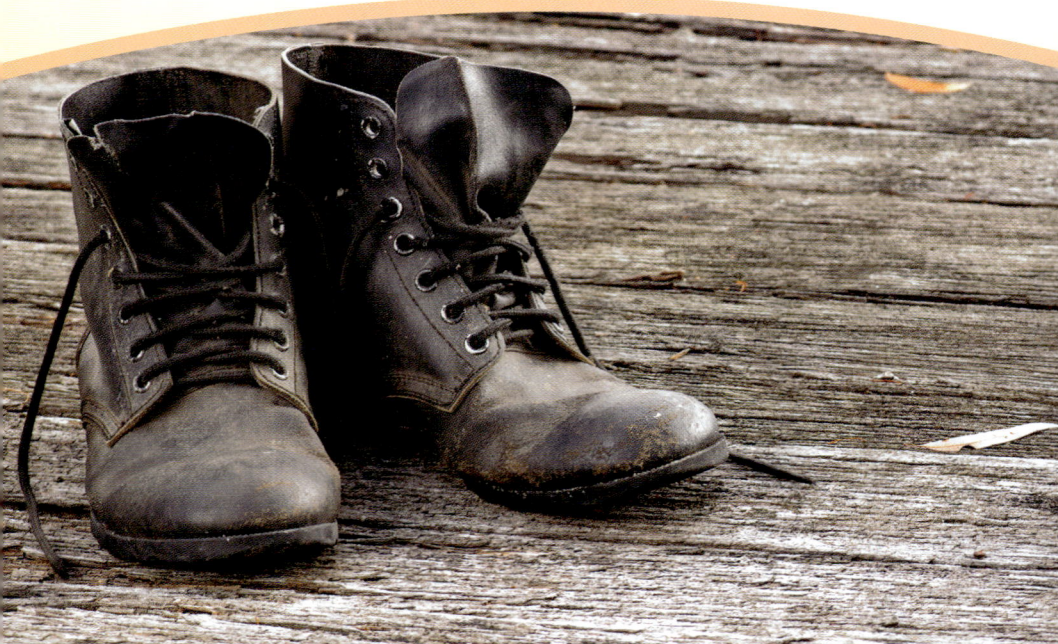

During his public ministry, Jesus had a much greater reputation for giving trustworthy, out-of-this-world "customer service." No one was ever ignored or neglected. He treated each one as if they were the only one. His warm, kindly gaze looked deeply into each person's heart in an attempt to understand their need. He could always be counted on to take time to listen and envelop hurting people in love.

The following are a few brief examples from the life of Christ that can help build our trust in him.

JESUS WELCOMES US

One of the most despised groups of people in all of Israel were the Jews who chose to collect taxes for Rome. Loose regulations allowed them to tax everything imaginable, usually extorting excessive fees to fill Roman coffers and pad their own bulging savings accounts. John MacArthur comments, "Most were despicable, vile, unprincipled scoundrels."[5]

Matthew, who later became a disciple of Jesus, was just such an individual. Against all odds, the savior asked him to become a leader in his new movement to change the world. Christ could not have chosen someone more hated by Jewish society. Despite people's rejection of Matthew, Jesus' only response was to find some way to draw him all the way into the center. It was an imperative for him, driven by a passion for inclusion for all individuals.

Matthew's joyful, incredulous response to such counterculture love was to throw a big scoundrel banquet at his oversized home for all of his fellow tax collectors and "other disreputable sinners" (Matt. 9:10). Jesus became the guest of honor.

When we come to Christ with all of our warts and failings, we can always trust that we will be made to feel that we belong. And we will be just as included when we come with our messes the millionth time as we were the first (see: Matthew 9:9–13; Mark 2:13–17; Luke 5:27–31).

> *He could always be counted on to take time to listen and envelop hurting people in love.*

JESUS UNDERSTANDS US

As I consider the ministry of Christ, I have to periodically remind myself that most of his life was spent as a blue-collar worker in a small-town carpenter shop. All we have to go on is a very brief reference in Matthew that records the derisive question, "Is not this the carpenter's son?" (Matt. 13:55, NKJV). That is enough, however, to open up a treasure trove of facts and images.

For over two decades, Jesus did manual labor in a very physically demanding profession. He sweat, stank, got splinters, blisters, and cuts, grunted, burped, strained, coughed from inhaled dust, ached, sneezed, and went home at night exhausted.

He had to know how to use an axe, adz, hatchet, saw, bow-drill, stone-headed hammer, wooden mallet, iron chisel, file, awl, and perhaps a plane for shaping wood.[6] He needed to be able to make farm tools, beams for home construction, door and window frames, tables, chairs, storage boxes, wooden carts and wheels, plows, winnowing forks, and other practical items.[7]

By his example, Jesus dignified work. He dignified doing daily chores. Whatever our tasks and burdens, Christ can be trusted to identify with our everyday struggles and understand our needs.

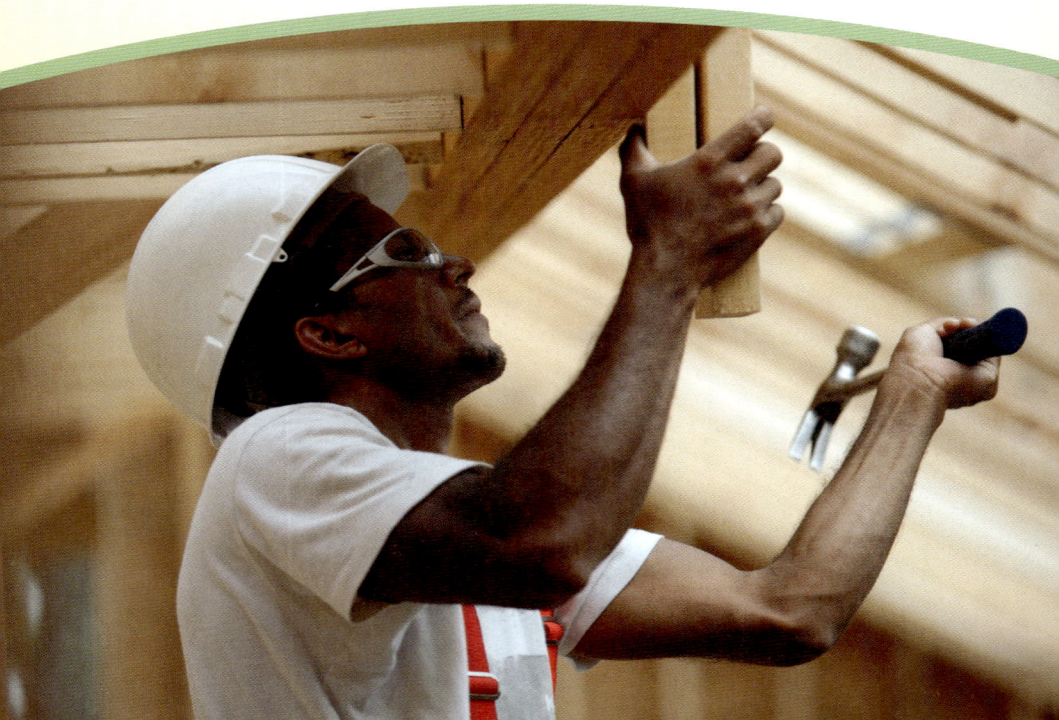

JESUS BEFRIENDS US

One of the most mind-blowing verses of Scripture regarding Jesus' insatiable desire to befriend everyone is found in Matthew. It takes us into the Garden of Gethsemane on the night of Christ's betrayal.

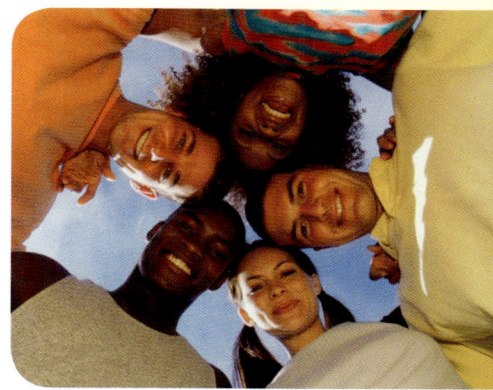

One of the twelve disciples, Judas, had already sold Jesus down the river for thirty pieces of silver. He then led the Lord's enemies to where Christ was spending the night so they could arrest him, put him on trial, and have him summarily executed. We read, "Now His betrayer had given them a sign, saying, 'Whomever I kiss, He is the One; seize Him.' Immediately he went up to Jesus and said, 'Greetings, Rabbi!' and kissed Him."

Now here comes the kicker, "But Jesus said to [Judas], '*Friend*, why have you come?'" (Matt. 26:48–50, NKJV, emphasis added).

Did you catch that? From all that our society teaches, there is no way that the word "friend" should be used in that sentence! I could see Jesus addressing his betrayer as "Informer," "Backstabber," "Traitor," "Turncoat," "Defector." Fully justified. But FRIEND? Absurd. Yet, there it is.

So what sense are we supposed to make of *that*? All I can conclude is that in Jesus' own heart, from his vantage point, *he had no enemies*. In his own mind, he refused to separate people into categories of good or bad, friends or enemies. He longed for everyone to be a friend, even though many didn't feel that way about him.

> *Whether we are rebelling against Christ and shaking our fist at him or worshipping him, he can be trusted to always relate to us as his very dear, close friend.*

JESUS SEES OUR HEART

Jesus was drained from engaging in rancorous debate with the Jewish authorities in an open area surrounding the Jewish Temple. The gospels tell us that he sat down to rest and hung his head. Eventually, Christ looked up and saw people putting donations in the nearby treasury receptacles. The funds were used for temple expenses.[8]

Some of the donors were quite wealthy. Painting the scene in modern terms, several well-groomed men in blue business suits stopped, pulled out their wallets, fingered their cash, and dropped in $500 to $1,000. Other well-to-do people paused, pulled out their checkbooks, and ceremoniously wrote out donations from $5,000 up.

Jesus' eyes suddenly locked onto a detail that took seconds to transpire but has been preserved in Scripture forever. During a lull in the activity, an elderly lady dressed in over-used, ragged clothing hurried up, dropped two pennies into the donation box, and scurried away. The savior followed her retreating form intently. His heart beat faster, like a father who had just watched his child hit a game-winning home run.

Deeply moved, Christ called out to the disciples, "Hey, guys, come over here quickly. You won't believe what I just saw. Absolutely amazing." He then related the events and concluded, "She gave more than all the others, a lot more."

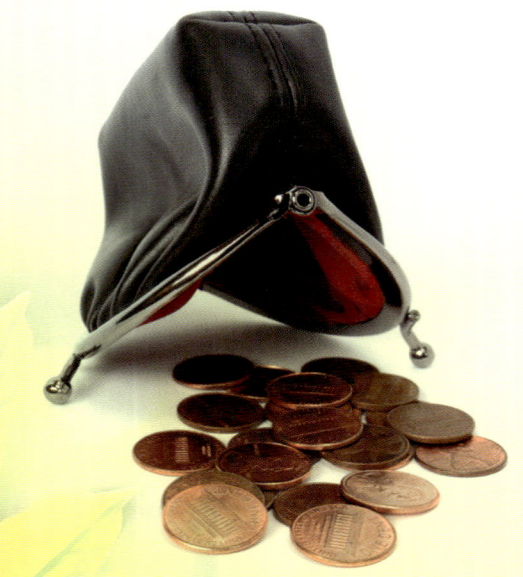

If you calculate based on amount, it was a pittance. But calculated based on *percentage*, it was mindboggling, because it was all she had – 100 percent. It wasn't really about money at all. It was about sacrifice and heart.[9]

How easily that incident could have passed into obscurity. But Jesus saw and made sure others knew.

With that story in mind, we can trust today that all of the little ways we give of ourselves to help others are highly valued by Christ. All of the anonymous ways we seek to lighten someone else's load at home, work, or in the community, all of the kind words shared that seem to evaporate into thin air once spoken, are all noticed by Jesus, and he is deeply, everlastingly moved (see Mark 12:41–44; Luke 21:1–4).

> *All of the anonymous ways we seek to lighten someone else's load are noticed by Jesus.*

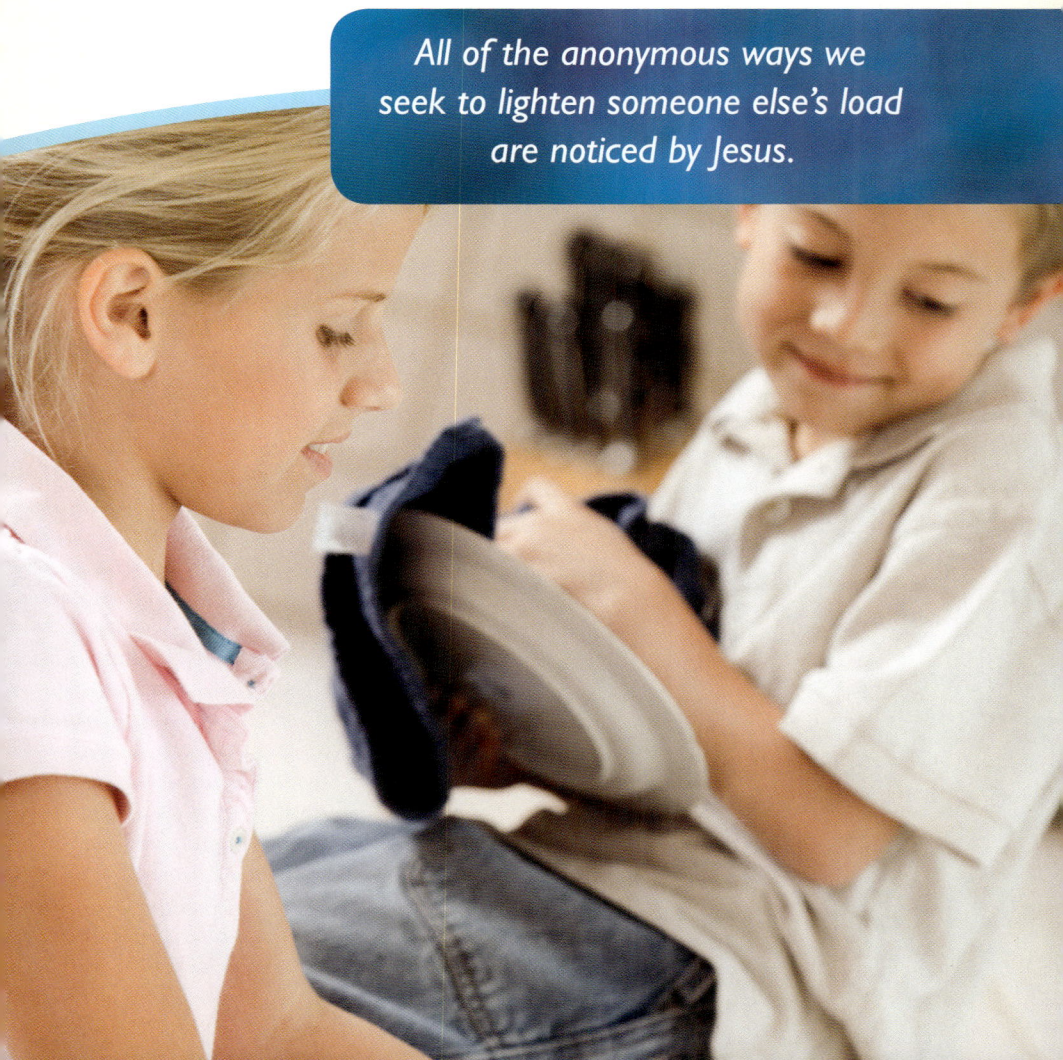

JESUS BREAKS DOWN BARRIERS

On the Monday before the crucifixion, Jesus was in the city of Jerusalem for the annual Feast of Passover. As he surveyed what was taking place at the Jewish Temple, anger stirred within him. Something had to be done.

Pilgrims by the tens of thousands from far and near jammed the streets of the holy city. Most were there to worship, which included paying a temple tax and offering an animal sacrifice. The tax had to be paid in the correct coinage, so booths were set up as a foreign exchange with a very hefty surcharge. Other booths sold animals at outrageous prices. The whole operation was a money-making machine.[10]

The buying and selling had turned the temple into a teeming marketplace with yelling, shouting, accusing, denouncing, not to mention the racket from thousands of livestock and birds. What angered Christ the most was that it all happened within what was called the Court of the Gentiles. This was the only place where Gentiles, non-Jews, could come to worship God and learn of him, and they were being deprived of that opportunity because of the bedlam.[11]

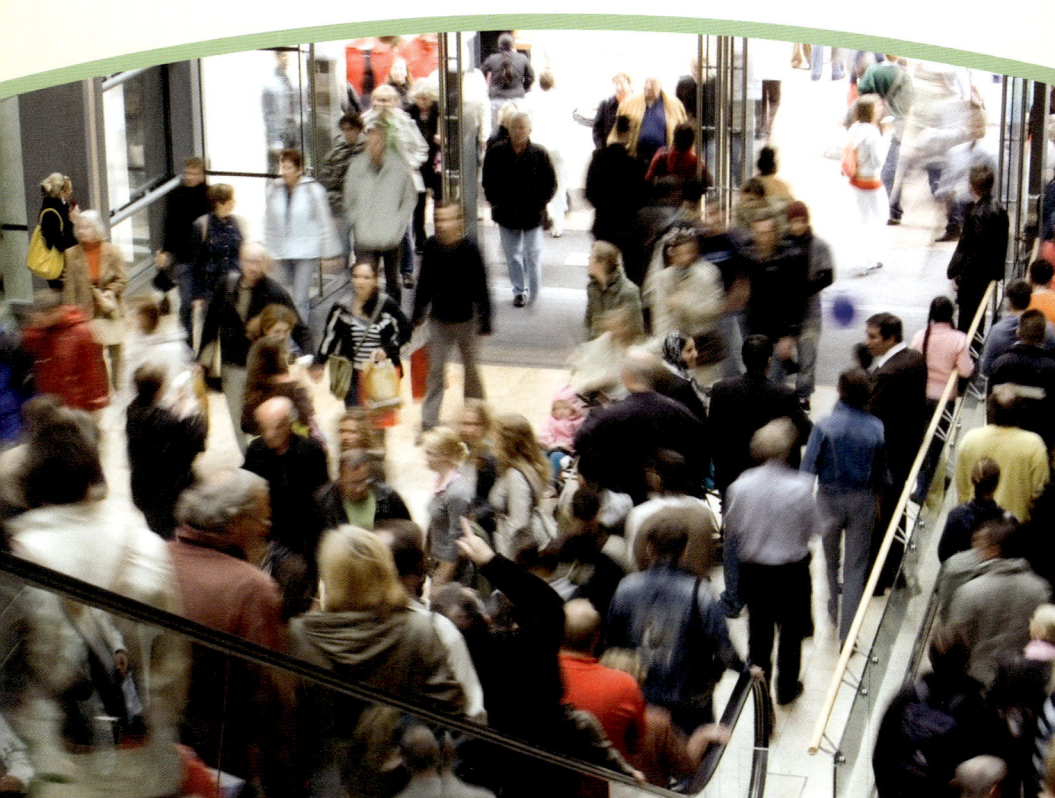

Nothing upsets Jesus more than something that is a barrier between us and him. The Gentiles were helpless to alter the situation, so Jesus decided to take charge. His eyes narrowed and his muscles tightened. He strode into the commotion and, with a carpenter's exceptional strength, upended tables, tossed cages, and flung money boxes. Hair flying, Christ single-handedly threw all of the merchants, thieves, and animals out, and there was finally quiet.

The Gentiles could, at last, worship God in peace. The barriers to knowing God had been completely removed. In the very next scene, little children are climbing up on Jesus' lap. What an amazing transformation!

For us today, we can trust that, if we ask him, Jesus will take the initiative to rid our lives of anything that in any way tends to separate us from him. The barrier may be a habit, an attitude, a sin, an emotional need, resentment, guilt, insecurity, a deep-seated feeling of doubt, or other issue. If we turn it over to Christ, he promises to bring resources into our lives, arrange circumstances, and guide our choices to eventually remove these hindrances. As he did for the Gentiles, he will do for us what we cannot do for ourselves. Our part is to surrender, trust, and follow his lead (see Matt. 21:12–16; Mark 11:15–19; Luke 19:45–48).

This short survey from the life of Christ is only a thought starter. It is only intended to point the way. Myriad other times Jesus demonstrated that he can, indeed, be trusted fully.

And in all these examples, we need to keep in mind the words of the disciple John, "No one has ever seen God. The only Son, who is the same as God and is at the Father's side, *he has made him known*" (John 1:18, GNT, emphasis added). If God the Father had been incarnated instead of Jesus, his earthly ministry would have unfolded in an equivalent way. If you've seen one, you've seen the other. If you have confidence in one, you can have confidence in the other. Christ established once and for all his own rock-solid trustworthiness and that of the Father as well.

DISCUSSION

Tell of a time when you experienced great customer service.

What does someone need to do to earn your trust?

In what ways would Jesus' call of Matthew have challenged the disciples?

How does it affect your understanding of God to know he spent many years making furniture and building houses?

What are some ways to turn an enemy into a friend?

What does it tell you about Jesus that he got excited about the woman's tiny offering?

Describe a spiritual or emotional barrier you are currently experiencing that you would like Jesus to get rid of.

Describe an experience from Jesus' ministry other than those mentioned in this lesson that helps establish his trustworthiness for you.

SHARING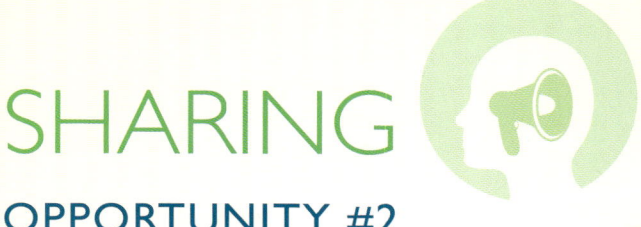

OPPORTUNITY #2

- Pray as a group for God to open the way for you to share something from these lessons to help someone else.

- Keep your radar up each day for opportunities.

ABUNDANT LIVING THOUGHT

When we come to Christ with all of our warts and failings, we can always trust that we will be made to feel that we belong.

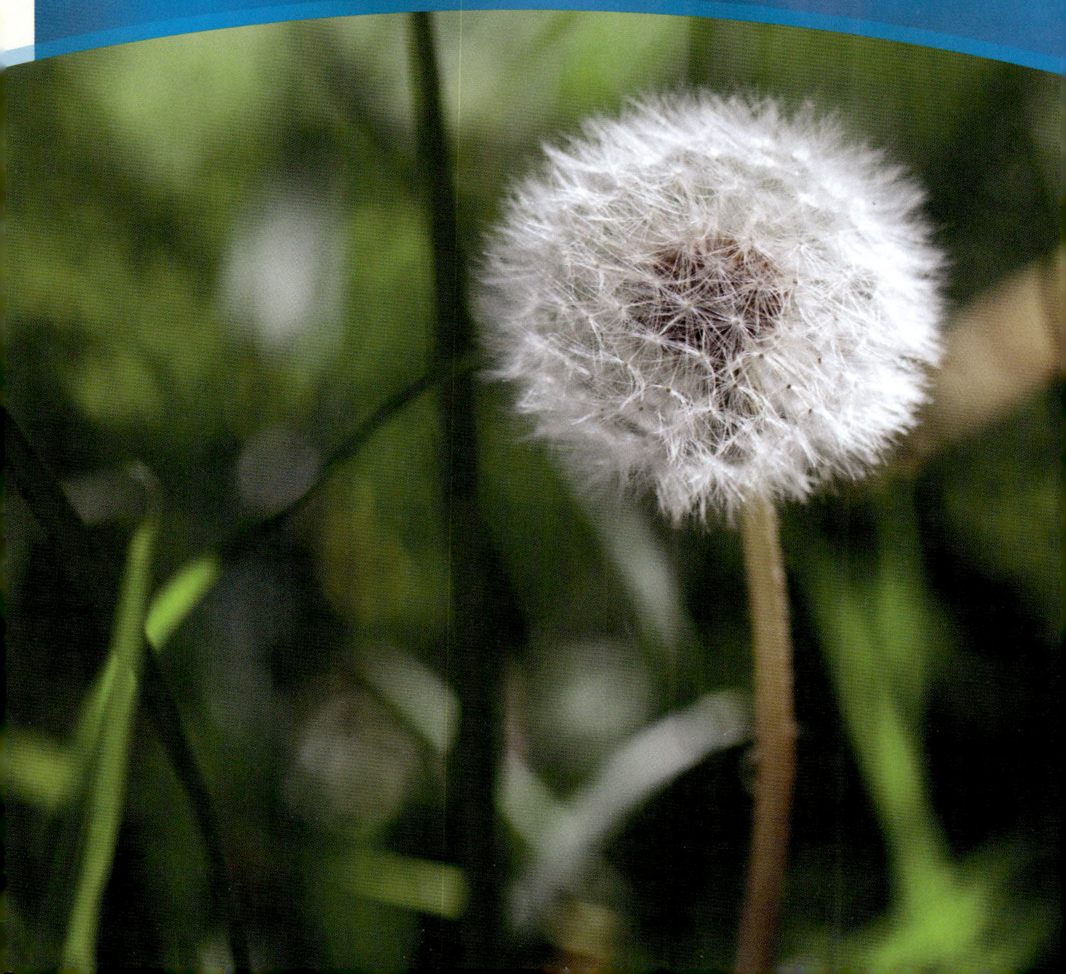

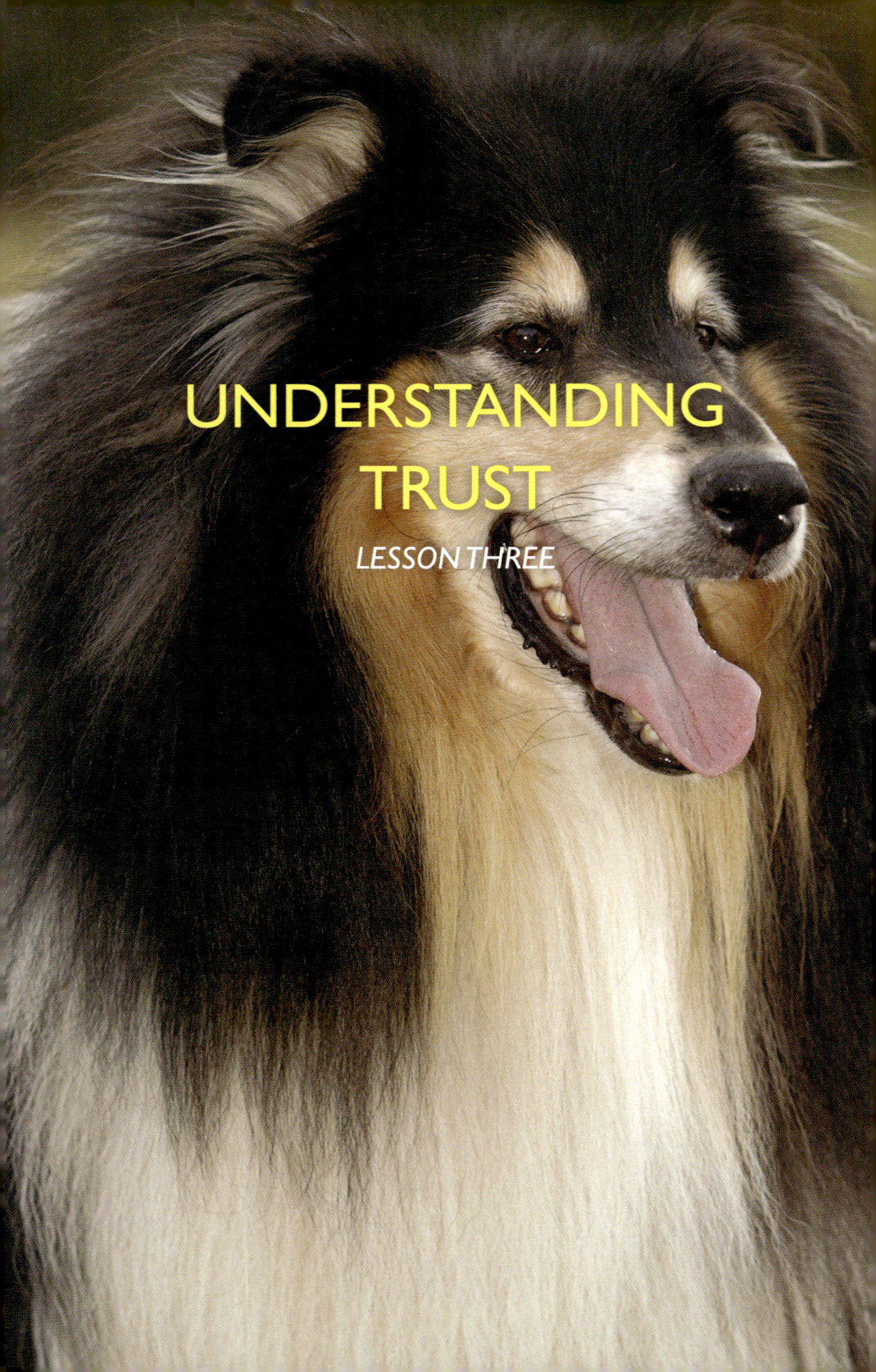

WARM UP

Feedback: In what ways did God open the door last week for you to share some part of the lesson with someone else?

....
....
....
....

Choose one or both questions to discuss (if in a group setting), or write out your answers on a separate sheet (for individual use):

1. **What things do you always make room for in your schedule besides work and family?**[12]

....
....
....

2. **Describe your favorite dessert.**

....
....
....

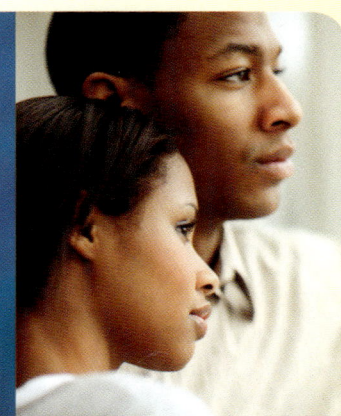

"A believer understands God can be trusted in all circumstances — even when it isn't clear why things happen the way they do."

GORDON RETZER

DISCOVERY

One afternoon, a driver on the New Jersey Turnpike was shocked at what he saw happen up ahead. While a Lincoln Town Car was traveling at full speed, the rear door opened and a passenger shoved a collie onto the pavement. The dog hit the concrete, rolled over several times, then landed in a ditch. Bleeding profusely, the collie got up and limped after the car and owner who had abandoned him so cruelly. Brennan Manning writes, "The dog's relentless faithfulness was not conditioned or diminished by the abuse and callous disregard of his master."[13]

The loyalty of the collie in this heartbreaking story captures the essence of God's attitude toward humanity. The Scriptures tell us that Jesus died for us, "while we were still sinners" (Romans 5:8, NIV). Even though mankind had rejected him, Christ's only thought was to continue to relentlessly pursue us by going to a cross on our behalf. Because the savior is so astonishingly and profoundly faithful to us, he is eminently worthy of our trust.

In order to respond appropriately, we need to know what kind of trust God expects from us. Jesus once asked, "When the Son of Man comes, will He really find faith on the earth?" (Luke 18:8, NKJV). He is not simply referring to the quantity of faith, but, more importantly, its *quality*. What sort of faith is the Son of God looking for? In this lesson we will explore the answer to that vital question by looking at various characteristics of biblical faith. We are treating the words "faith" and "trust" as essentially synonymous.[14]

TRUST IN A PERSON

God certainly wants us to trust in Scripture and the information it contains. But more than that, we are invited to put our trust in the author of that information, the Son of God. The apostle Paul wrote, "God puts people right through their faith in Jesus Christ" (Rom. 3:22, GNT). It takes a powerful person whose heart beats with infinite love to provide us with the new life we need for daily living and the hope we need for the future. The carpenter from Nazareth, the flesh and blood human who is also fully divine, is just that kind of person. It is in his character, his caring, his ability, that we place our confidence and trust. Salvation is personal. It is a relationship.

TRUST IS A GIFT

The kind of trust that Christ is looking for cannot be self-generated. Our sinful, insecure hearts are not capable of producing it. We cannot grit our teeth and make ourselves trust. Like everything else in the spiritual life, it has to be a gift from our redeemer. Notice the following two verses from the pen of the apostle Paul:

> *For I say, through the grace given to me, to everyone who is among you, not to think of himself more highly than he ought to think, but to think soberly,* as God has dealt to each one a measure of faith *(Rom. 12:3, NKJV, emphasis added).*

> *Looking unto Jesus,* the author and finisher of our faith, *who for the joy that was set before Him endured the cross, despising the shame, and has sat down at the right hand of the throne of God (Hebrews 12:2, NKJV, emphasis added).*

Paul knew from experience that he could not have created his own trust in God from within himself. It had to be "authored" from the outside, from a divine source. We can nurture trust, but only God can place it within us to begin with. We can grow God's gift and deepen it through Bible study, prayer, and exercising faith, but we cannot originate it.

> *We can nurture trust, but only God can place it within us to begin with.*

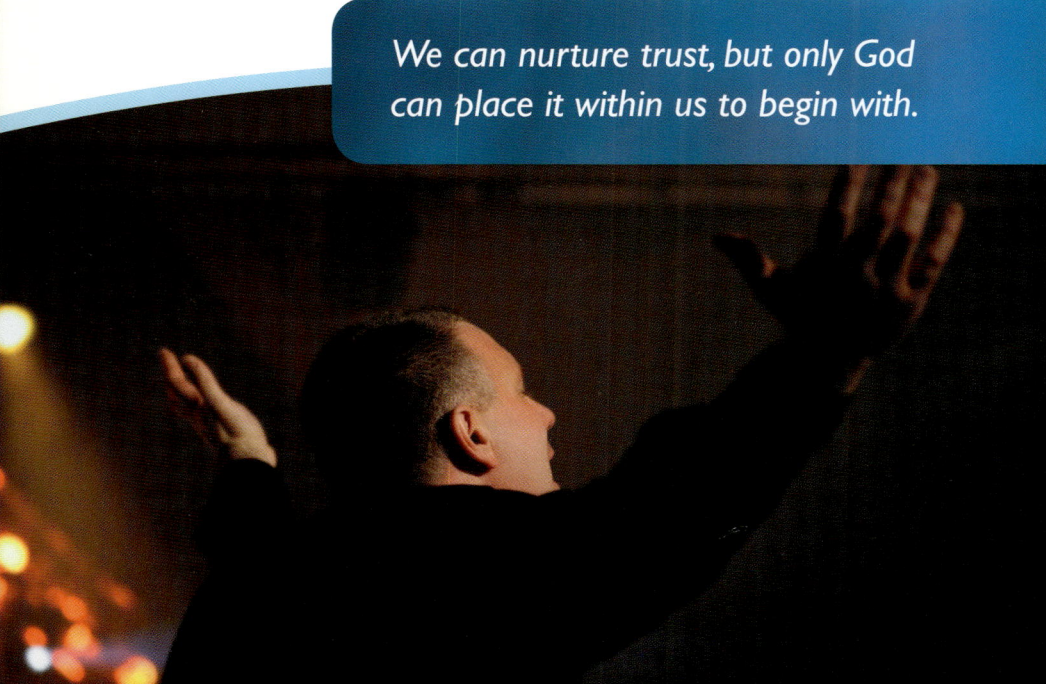

TRUST IS AN ALTERNATE WAY OF SEEING

The Scriptures give us the following definition of faith: "Faith is the confidence that what we hope for will actually happen; it gives us assurance about things we cannot see" (Heb. 11:1).

Trust in God is a way of perceiving that transcends physical sight. It makes what we hope for so real that it actually conditions the way we live. Faith brings unseen spiritual realities into such clear focus that we talk about them as if they were visible. It is not a fanciful way of seeing, but an alternative one.

Science has developed special goggles that enable people to see someone two hundred yards away on a pitch black, moonless, cloudy night. One way the technology operates is to capture the infrared light emitted by the heat from the person's body. Without those goggles, the person is invisible to the human eye.[15]

Trust in God is like those goggles. It enables us to perceive realities that are not visible to people who choose not to trust.

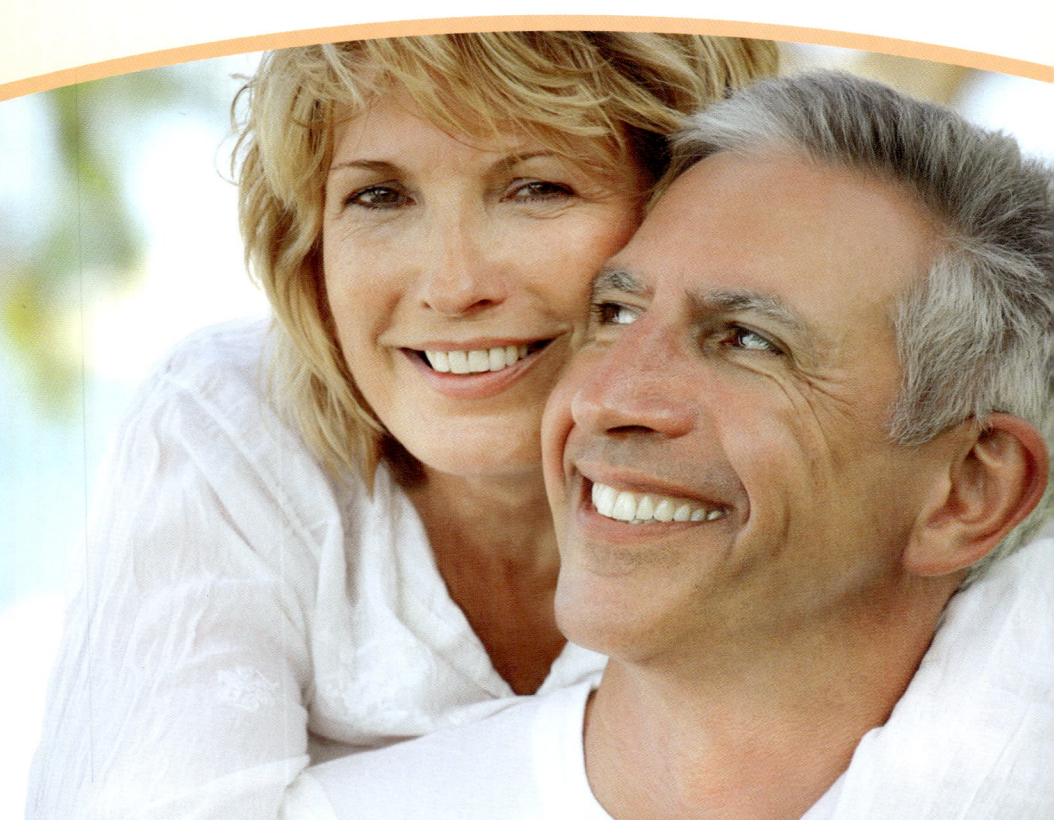

TRUST AND DOUBT

I wish someone had told me years ago that it's OK for a Christian to doubt spiritual things. Trust and doubt are normal elements of our religious journey. By "doubt" I don't mean shaking my fist at God in open rebellion. I mean those periodic potholes on the road of faith that cause us to question and re-examine our own thinking.

It is unrealistic to think that someone can maintain perfect trust in God in all circumstances without periods of doubt. The presence of doubting thoughts does not mean we are losing our spiritual grip. It simply means that we are human. Trust in God does not come naturally to humanity, and sometimes we will feel the tug of our old disbelieving self. Doubt can be a signal that we are weary, angry, or discouraged and need to take time to renew. Doubt can cause us to search deeper. Doubt can provide an opportunity to consciously reaffirm our faith.

Jesus once commented, "Assuredly, I say to you, among those born of women there has not risen one greater than John the Baptist" (Matt. 11:11, NKJV). That pretty much puts John at the pinnacle of the pantheon of great Christians. And yet, at one point, John was also assaulted by doubt. As he languished in prison, the devil bombarded him with questions regarding Jesus' role as Messiah. The depressed captive sent the following message through his followers, asking Christ, "Are You the Coming One, or do we look for another?" (Luke 7:19, NKJV).

Jesus knew John's heart. He saw the big picture of his life. He understood what a struggle it can sometimes be to trust and sent back a compassionate reply that restored John's hope and courage (see Luke 7:22–23).

Trust in God is a way of perceiving that transcends physical sight. It makes what we hope for so real that it actually conditions the way we live.

TRUST AND FEELINGS

Trust is boosted and comforted by warm feelings, but it is not dependent on them. It is wonderful when feelings of assurance wash over me in my Christian journey, but I don't depend on those feelings as an indicator that my spiritual walk is genuine and authentic. In fact, the purest form of trust in God probably occurs when our feelings run dry.

It has been helpful for me to think of three key words in this regard: fact, faith, and feeling. They are like a short train, with fact as the locomotive, faith as the passenger car, and feeling as the caboose. Even if the caboose drops away, the passenger car can still get to its destination as long as it stays connected to the locomotive.

The facts are the promises and truths of God's Word. Faith is our willingness to trust those facts. Feelings may or may not tag along. Feelings are fickle and can often run contrary. They are usually an unreliable barometer of our true experience. You may feel like God is not present, like you are not progressing spiritually, like you are battling on your own. That is when you need to *choose to trust* in the truths of Scripture that say otherwise, regardless of how you feel.

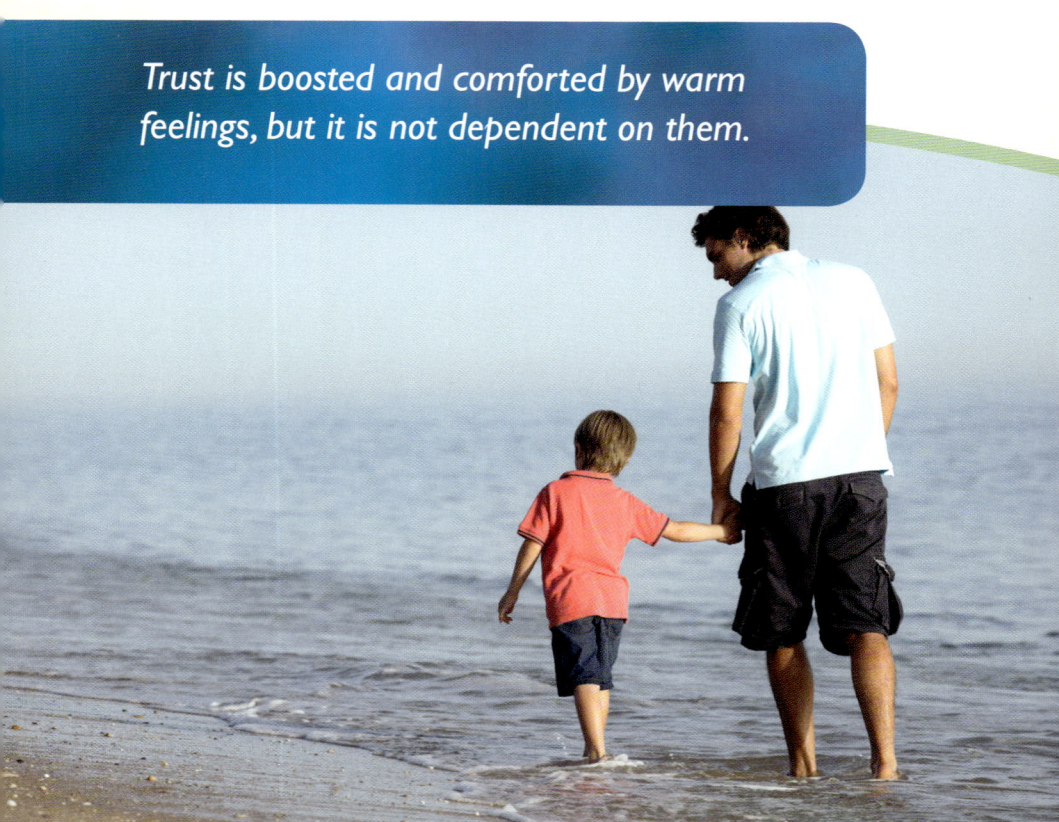

Trust is boosted and comforted by warm feelings, but it is not dependent on them.

DIFFICULTIES TRUSTING

My dad was an alcoholic. He had many good qualities, but they were all overshadowed when he hit the bottle. Good dad became belligerent, mean, disrespectful, obnoxious dad – especially on weekends.

He and I were very close. Being excessively shy as a child, I would spend weekends doing things with him rather than with the kids from the neighborhood. I lived for the weekends. Too often we'd be headed back from an errand and he'd stop at the liquor store or bar. The bar was the worst because I'd get left in the car alone for what seemed like forever. I was terrified by the thoughts: *Is he OK? Will he be coming back?*

When he did finally return, I knew what to expect. His eyes would be glazed over, his speech would be slurred, and the weekend would be ruined. Over time, my trust in Dad was severely eroded from repeated disappointments.

As a typical ACOA (Adult Children Of Alcoholics), I have had difficulty throughout my adult life trusting others. My trust can be too hard to win and too easy to lose. I often hesitate to allow my hopes to get too high for fear they might be dashed. There are, of course, many types and degrees of neglect and abuse suffered by both children and adults, and many have trust issues far worse than mine.

All of this has important implications for one's spiritual journey. I have come to understand that people are not like light switches. You cannot be raised to distrust and then suddenly switch to trusting because it now involves God. It takes time. It takes trial and error and tremendous courage. It can mean taking three steps forward and one or two back. But it can get better, a lot better.

Through my wife's love, the support of friends, and the insights of Christian counselors, I have shed many mental and emotional misconceptions. I also find great assurance in Jesus' promise to be always with me (Matt. 28:20). I have come to trust the apostle Paul's statement that Christ is steadfast, the same yesterday, today, forever (Heb. 13:8, NIV). I still need to be alert to the lurking presence of old perspectives. But I strive, by God's grace, to look beyond them to know the truth about how trustworthy God really is.

TRUSTING IN SPITE OF DISTORTIONS

One of the main hindrances to trusting God is the distorting influence of society's values and priorities. We swim in a sea of un-God-like norms and behaviors. What is utterly abnormal to him has become very normal to humanity in general.

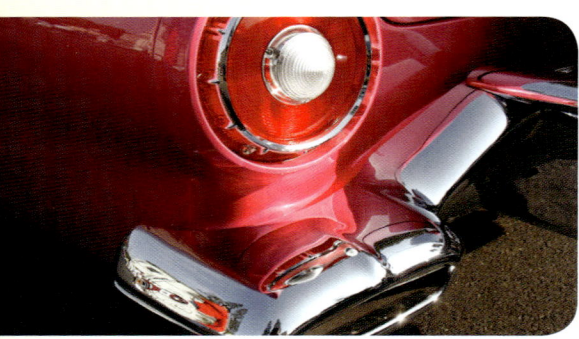

The way many people treat each other is not the way he wants to relate to us. The real danger comes when we project warped elements of life on earth onto God. And whenever our view of him becomes distorted by wrong comparisons, it makes it harder to trust.

The apostle Paul put it this way, "For now we see in a mirror, dimly, but then face to face. Now I know in part, but then I shall know just as I also am known" (1 Cor. 13:12, NKJV). Ancient mirrors only allowed you to see yourself "dimly," as Paul puts it. It was like looking at your reflection in the fender of your car. I can imagine Paul gazing into the mirror of his day, squinting, turning the device this way and that, trying to discern what he really looked like.

It's like that, the apostle says, in trying to see God. We strain to grasp his true character. We catch helpful insights into what he is truly like, but huge gaps can remain. Acknowledging that potential gaps and distortions exist puts us on guard and helps us realize that problems in our spiritual life often have their root in our misconceptions regarding God. Identifying these distortions can free us and provide a kind of corrective spiritual lens.

> *God's love has no conditions.*
> *His love shines on us*
> *continuously like the sun.*

A few examples of the contrast between our world and God's:

- Apart from God, society can only produce counterfeit love. It is conditional, what I call, "I love you IF." When the loved one doesn't live up to expectations, the affection is removed. In stark contrast, God's love has no conditions. His love shines on us continuously like the sun.

- Society says we get what we deserve. In God's kingdom, we get what we *don't* deserve.

- Society says we are valuable when we are smart, beautiful/handsome, and successful. From God's perspective, each of us is of infinite worth, period. Worth is a gift. There are no prerequisites, no qualifications, nothing to measure up to.

- Society is built upon a hierarchy with the lowest classes serving those above them. In the spiritual realm, the greatest serve the lowest and the weakest. Jesus said, "But he who is greatest among you shall be your servant" (Matt. 23:11, NKJV). God leads by serving. He always puts our needs first.

Distortions cloud our perception of God's love and, as a result, have the potential of damaging or limiting our trust in him. Only through careful study of the truth about God as revealed in Scripture can we see through those distortions and consistently trust the One who is so incredibly trustworthy.

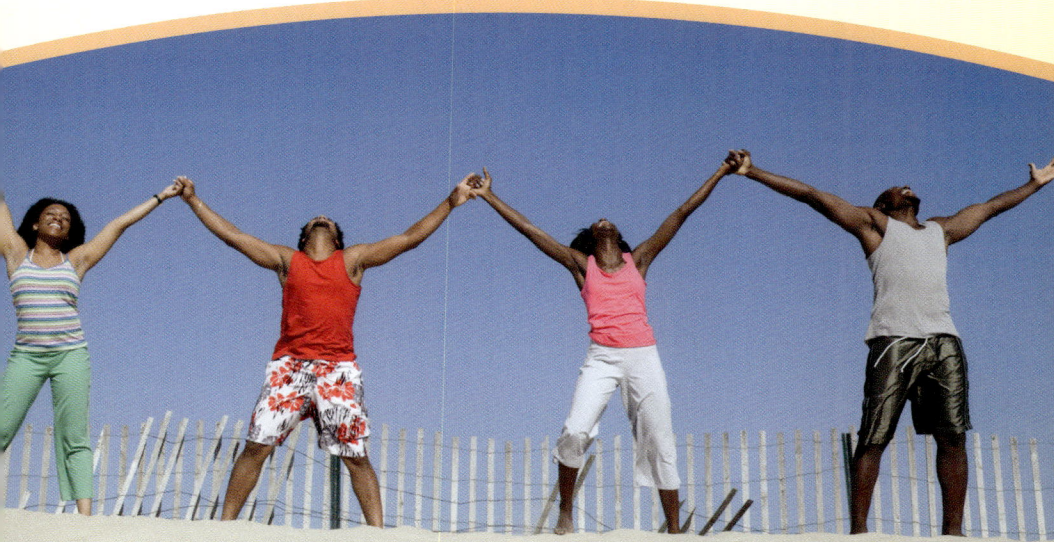

DISCUSSION

What is the difference between *trust* and *belief*? Give an example.

What is the difference between *knowing about* Jesus and *trusting in him*?

If trust in God is a gift, what is our part in nurturing it? What are some ways to do that?

What would you say to someone who told you they doubt God cares about them?

What helps you the most to connect with God when he feels like he is a million miles away?

What experiences from your past might undermine your ability to trust God as much as you would like?

Describe a time when you got something you didn't deserve. What window does that open into the heart of God?

How has your sense of self-worth changed over the years?

SHARING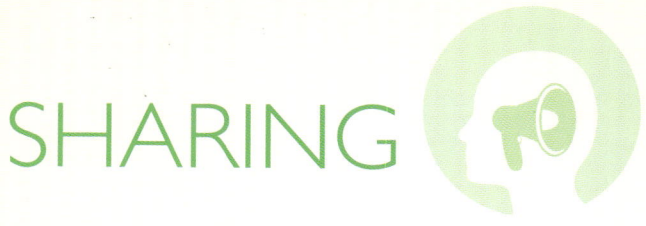

OPPORTUNITY #3:

- Pray as a group for God to open the way for you to share something from these lessons to help someone else this week.
- Keep your radar up each day for opportunities.

ABUNDANT LIVING THOUGHT

From God's perspective, each of us is of infinite worth. Such worth is a gift. There are no prerequisites, no qualifications, nothing to measure up to.

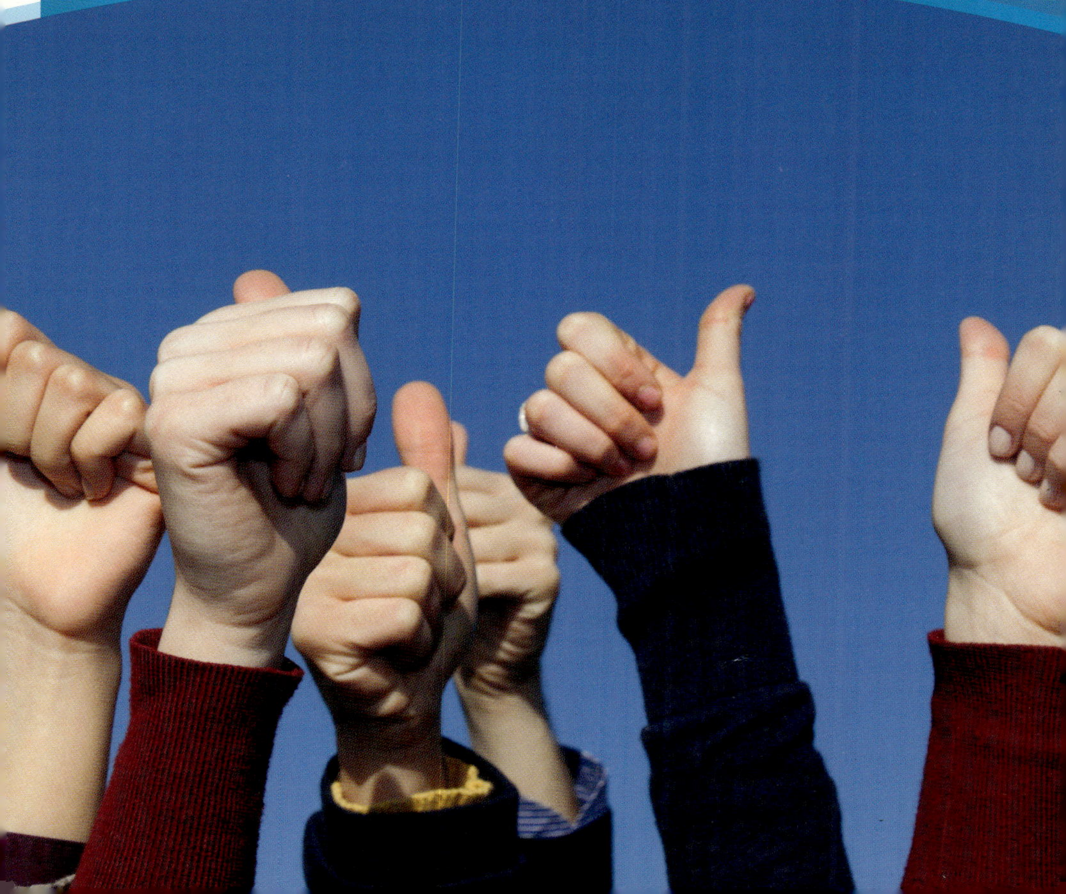

TRUSTING GOD FOR NEW LIFE

LESSON FOUR

WARM UP

Feedback: In what ways did God open the door last week for you to share some part of the lesson with someone else?

....
....
....
....

Choose one or both questions to discuss (if in a group setting), or write out your answers on a separate sheet (for individual use):

1. **Have you ever had a nickname? Where did it come from?**

....
....
....

2. **What old friend would you like to contact that you haven't seen in many years? Why would you like to contact them?**[16]

....
....
....

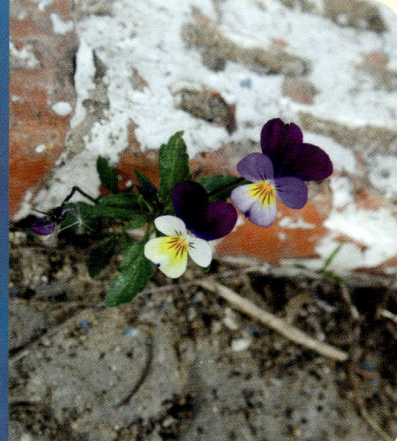

"When we trust in God we are transformed from people of fear to people of courage — and from people of courage to people of purpose."

DR. DES CUMMINGS JR.

DISCOVERY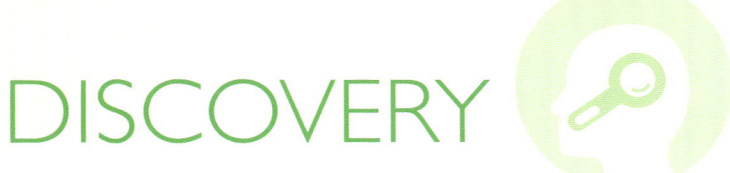

Ethan noticed the small discolored patch of skin on the upper portion of his right shoulder during his morning bath. A frightening image instantly flashed through his mind. The voice of his wife Joanna calling everyone to breakfast pulled his thoughts back to the pressing duties of the day.

The couple's two teenage sons and nine-year-old daughter hurried to join the simple morning meal. The disjointed conversation focused mainly on the oppressively hot weather and last night's homework assignments. Running late, Ethan excused himself before finishing, grabbed a hunk of crusty homemade bread, and headed out the door to his job as a metal worker.

Thanks to steady contracts from the government, Ethan had enough income for the couple to purchase their own home and live comfortably. He had originally apprenticed under one of the best craftsmen in the region and now had enough experience and respect from his peers to mentor others.

Several relatives lived nearby, including both parents, two uncles, and Joanna's grandmother. Weekends were often filled with visits and shared meals. Storytelling and laughter created a warm, reassuring atmosphere.

Ethan now monitored the discolored patch on a daily basis, and his heart shuddered as he watched it grow significantly. He chose to not say anything yet to Joanna. He had a hard time sleeping and paying attention at work. Over the next several weeks other patches appeared, with one eventually showing up on the left side of his forehead that was impossible to hide.

Joanna inquired nervously. Tearfully, she and Ethan shared their suspicions and fears with each other in hushed conversations. Others soon noticed as well. Local authorities were informed. A physical examination ensued. All too quickly the diagnosis came back – leprosy.

Within the hour, officials ordered Ethan to leave the village by himself and take up residence for the rest of his life in a quarantined leper colony about thirty miles away. Joanna was inconsolable. The children were in utter shock and bewilderment. Would they ever see their dad again? How could the family survive financially? In an instant, the future was destroyed.

Ethan could not enter any town, could not come in contact with any non-lepers, could not attend the worship services that he loved, and could no longer pursue his career. Such were the Jewish laws in the days of Christ. In Bible times, leprosy was untreatable.[17]

Life in the leper colony was a constant struggle, being surrounded by constant reminders of what he would one day become. As weeks grew into years, Ethan's body and spirit were eaten up more and more by the disease until he became utterly disgusting even to himself.

That story is imagined, but it was all too typical in New Testament times. Ethan's experience could easily have been the background of the desperate leper who, against all odds, came one momentous day into Jesus' presence, yelling for help. Like Ethan, he had been banished from home and taken up residence far from all that he held dear.

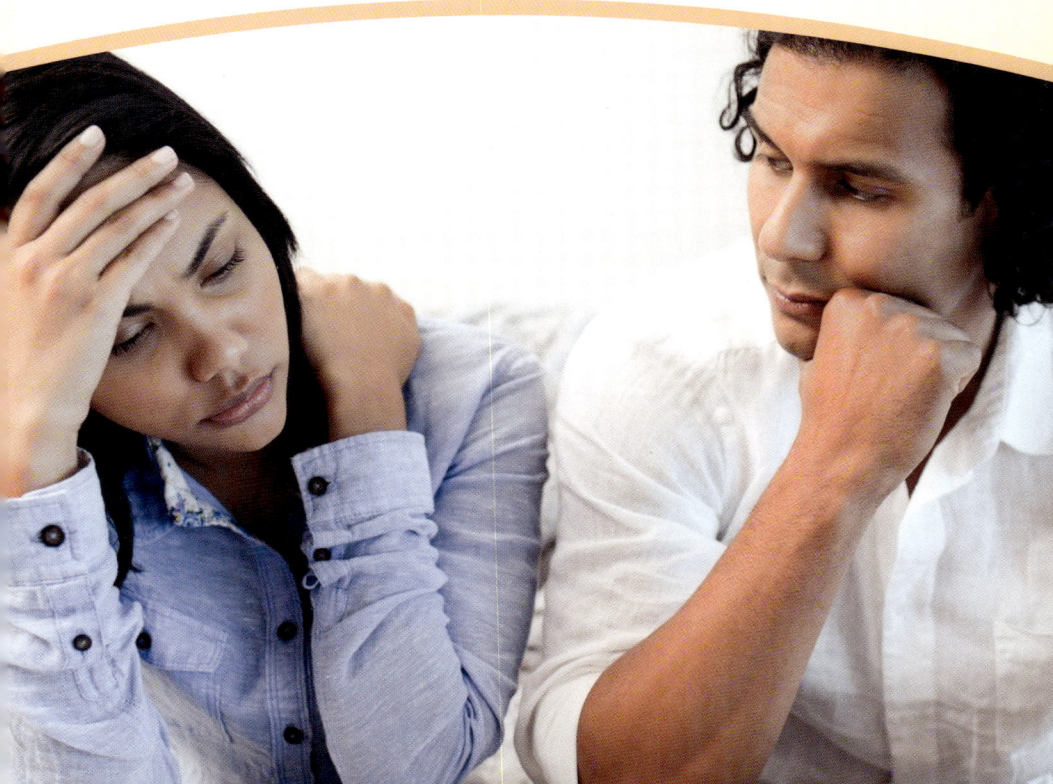

The Gospel of Luke reports that he was "full of leprosy" (Luke 5:12, KJV). An advanced case, he was most likely covered with rotting flesh and ulcerating sores, oozing a foul-smelling liquid.[18] We read that the poor man bowed before Christ, tearfully begging for assistance.

In response, the first thing Jesus did was to provide inner healing of the man's spirit. Matthew's gospel tells us that Christ, in a remarkable gesture of caring, broke strict religious regulations and *touched him* before he healed him physically (Matt. 8:3). The Son of God gently placed his palm directly onto those awful, running sores and tenderly wrapped his thick carpenter fingers around the man's deteriorating shoulder. Knowing that the victim had not felt a human touch for years, the savior focused initially on spiritual and emotional restoration. It was a touch of deep empathy and unconditional acceptance designed to restore the victim's devastated sense of self-worth. It was an unheard-of gesture of friendship and concern.

It is vital to understand that Jesus accepted the man before he was acceptable, while he was still riddled with the disease. There was nothing the man could do to earn that acceptance. It was a 100 percent gift from the heart of our redeemer. All the leper could do was to come and admit his need.

After providing the gift of acceptance, Jesus then got rid of the leprosy itself. He replaced any missing fingers or toes. He turned the myriad lesions into skin as smooth and healthy as that of a little child. In my imagination I can see the former leper giving Christ a long, tearful hug, then running home and joyously renewing long-lost relationships with his beloved family and friends.

> *It is vital to understand that Jesus accepted the man before he was acceptable.*

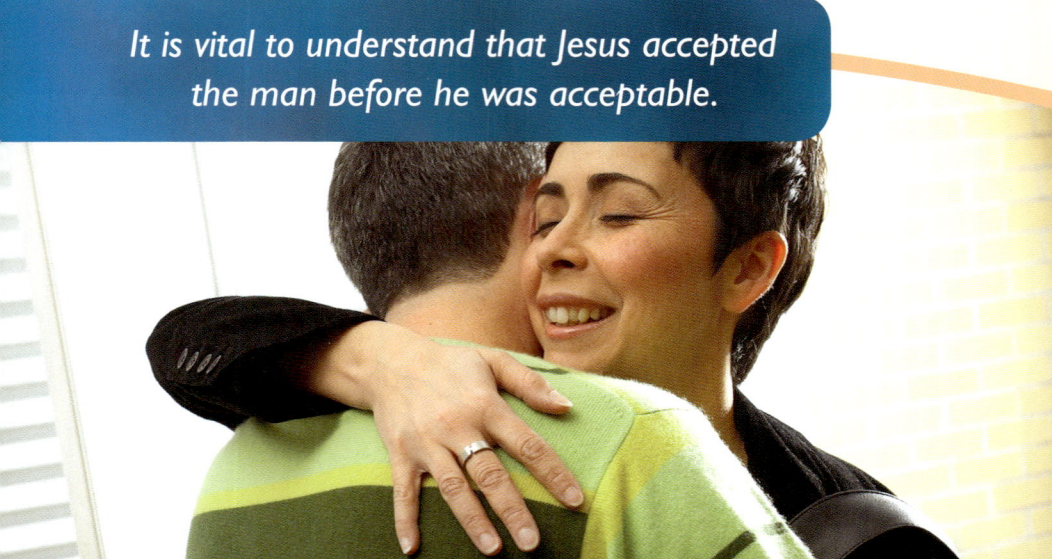

In the Old Testament, the prophet Isaiah uses leprosy to describe our spiritual condition, "The whole head is sick, and the whole heart faint. From the sole of the foot even unto the head there is no soundness in it; but wounds, and bruises, and putrifying sores" (Isa. 1:5–6, KJV).

We are infected with the disease of sin that destroys our hopes and derails our happiness. It is a spiritual illness that has corrupted our motives and transformed us from being God-centered to being fundamentally centered on self.

Like he did for the leper during his public ministry, Jesus wants to provide us with new life today. He is anxious to give us forgiveness and eternal life. He longs to touch us with acceptance and rid us of the debilitating effects of sin. He will marshal all the resources of heaven to make sure our spiritual leprosy is cured.

So how can we receive these marvelous gifts? What should our response be to such underserved generosity and love? It all boils down to trust.

1. God's Perspective.

First we need to trust that God's estimation of our spiritual condition is, in fact, true. We have to admit our need and be willing for him to change us from the inside out.

Imagine a horribly disfigured leper who refuses to admit his actual circumstance:

> Jesus – "So, how are you doing?"
>
> Leper – "Not bad really. Getting along just fine, thank-you. Rarely felt better."
>
> Jesus – "But what about all those wounds and sores? Those missing fingers and toes? That can't be good."
>
> Leper – "To tell you the truth, it doesn't really bother me all that much. Hardly notice it on most days."

That makes no sense, especially considering all that Jesus has to offer. But some people can be like that when it comes to salvation. "I'm not in bad shape spiritually, thank-you. Doing just fine really." But the apostle Paul gave humanity a vital reality check when he wrote, "For all have sinned and fall short of the glory of God" (Rom. 3:23, NKJV). Like the leper, unless we admit our need, we will keep ourselves at arms' length from divine assistance and joy.

2. God's Acceptance.

Once we decide to trust Jesus' evaluation of our helpless spiritual condition, we then need to trust that he accepts us *just as we are*. He accepts us before we are acceptable, with all of our faults and failings. As we kneel before him, longing for something better, we suddenly sense his wonderful restorative touch. It is at that moment that we are given the priceless gift of forgiveness and salvation. In that very instant, we have eternal life.

Unfortunately, many individuals know about Christ and do their best to follow his teachings, but they never feel assured of their eternal destiny. They think that it would be too audacious or presumptuous of them to believe they have salvation. The gospel writer John had something to say about such spiritual insecurity. In the little letter of 1 John, he records, "I write these things to you who believe in the name of the Son of God so *that you may know that you have eternal life*" (1 John 5:13, NIV, emphasis added).

John wanted his readers to be sure of their future. He understood that God wants us to have confidence that we are members of his family and is pained by our uncertainty. How would I feel if you asked my daughter if she was a member of our family and she replied, "Hope so." Hope so! I would feel terrible if she gave an answer like that, and God feels the same way about us.

Uncertainty usually betrays an underlying feeling that we aren't good enough to be saved when, in fact, we can never be good enough. The apostle Paul provides a wonderful answer to that misunderstanding when he writes, "Saving is all [God's] idea, and all his work. All we do is trust him enough to let him do it. It's God's gift from start to finish!" (Eph. 2:8–10, MSG).

That assurance is ours as long as we stay connected to God. When we commit our lives to him, it is like getting married. Every marriage has normal ups and downs, joys and challenges. But the marriage is still in place unless the relationship is dissolved through persistent, ongoing neglect or a divorce. So it is in the spiritual realm. Falling on our face spiritually does not cancel our salvation any more than an argument cancels a marriage. We learn from our mistakes, ask for forgiveness, and carry on. As long as our marriage to Jesus is alive and intact, our assurance remains.

It is reassuring to know that Jesus will exert the same tenaciousness in keeping the relationship together as he did in pursuing us in the first place. He will make it as easy as possible for us to stay close and as difficult as possible for us to stray away. During his ministry he declared, "And I give unto them eternal life; and they shall never perish, neither shall any man pluck them out of my hand" (John 10:28, KJV).

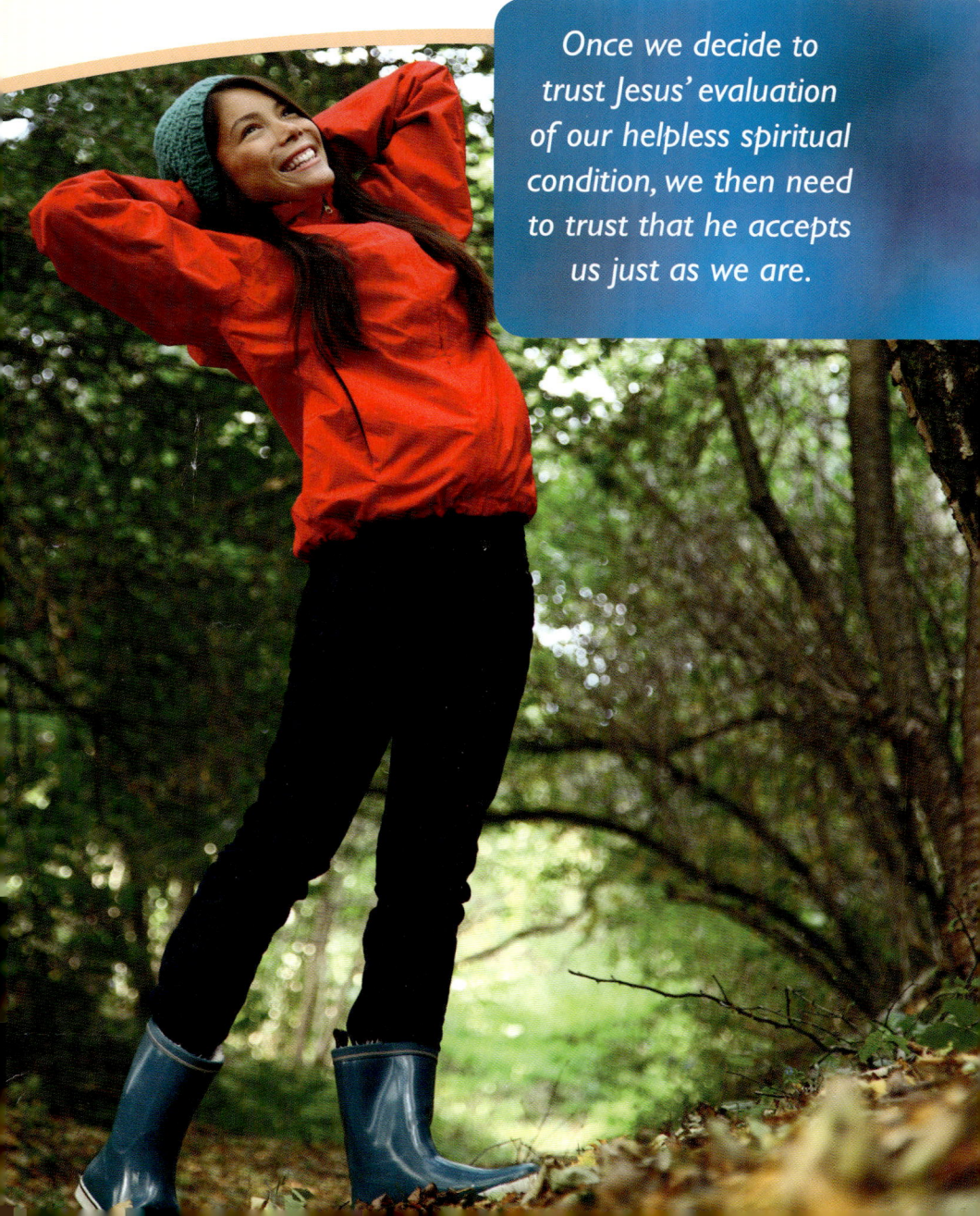

Once we decide to trust Jesus' evaluation of our helpless spiritual condition, we then need to trust that he accepts us just as we are.

3. God's Transforming Power.

We now go a step further. After the leper in the gospel story experienced Jesus' total acceptance, he needed to allow himself to be healed of the leprosy itself. He needed total regeneration.

So it is with us spiritually. God wants us not only to be forgiven but also to be transformed. Once we have the assurance of salvation through faith in Jesus Christ, we then need to trust God for an infusion of new life for daily living. God doesn't simply forgive us and leave us to struggle on without him. At the very moment we receive Jesus' saving touch, he moves in and takes up residence within our hearts through the powerful working of his Holy Spirit. He begins the lifelong work of remodeling our motives and reshaping our desires.

Think of the following verses as a promise to you personally. They speak of God's power to remake us so we can experience life to the fullest:

> *Because God is always at work in you to make you willing and able to obey his own purpose (Phil. 2:13, GNT).*
>
> *Anyone who is joined to Christ is a new being; the old is gone, the new has come (2 Cor. 5:17, GNT).*
>
> *For we are God's masterpiece. He has created us anew in Christ Jesus, so we can do the good things he planned for us long ago (Eph. 2:10).*
>
> *If we confess our sins, He is faithful and just to forgive us our sins and to* cleanse us from all unrighteousness *(1 John 1:9, NKJV, emphasis added).*

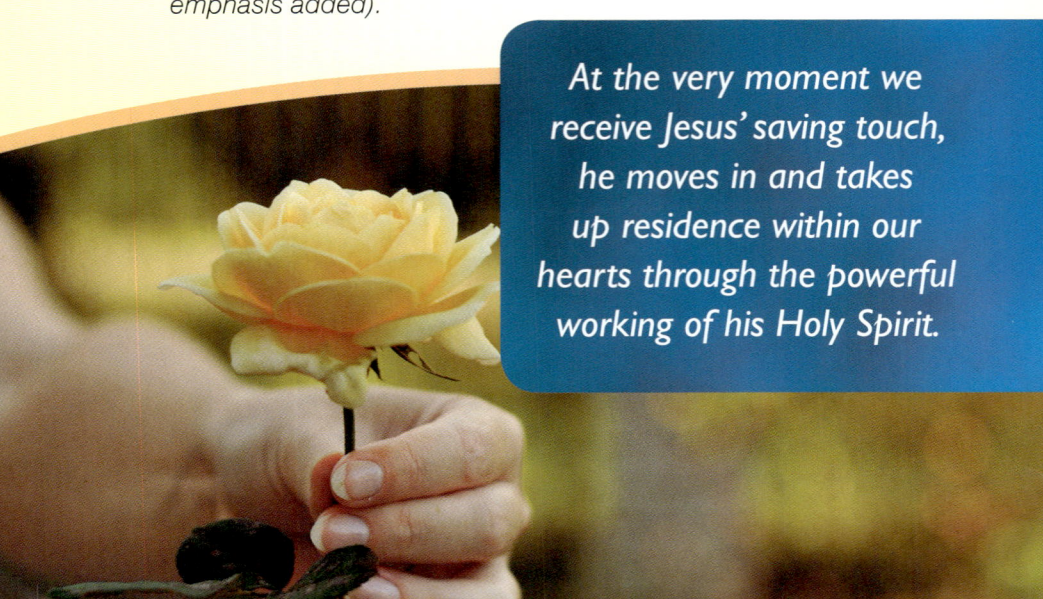

> *At the very moment we receive Jesus' saving touch, he moves in and takes up residence within our hearts through the powerful working of his Holy Spirit.*

Imagine that a man who is going in for gallbladder surgery has a hard time trusting his doctor. They give him a local anesthetic so he is awake during the entire procedure. He maintains a distrustful running commentary:

> *"You people all trained properly? Got good grades and everything? Top of your class?"*

> *"You know I'm in here for my gallbladder, don't you? I don't want you messing with any other organs."*

> *"Did you sterilize everything real good? If there's somebody else's germs on those tools it could be curtains for me. You realize that, don't you?"*

> *"Hey, shouldn't you be making that incision more to the left?"*

> *"There's way too much bleeding going on down there! Look at you guys with my blood all over your hands. That can't be good! Close me up!"*

> *"Hey, that doesn't look like a gallbladder to me. Put that thing back in there."*

> *"Don't touch that. Leave that alone."*

On and on, all due to a lack of trust.

So it is with us and Jesus, the great physician. He can operate with great expertise, but we have to cooperate by trusting and yielding control on an ongoing basis. The only effective way to maintain such trust is to continually deepen our relationship with the one who is so incredibly trustworthy. Christ described the dynamic this way, "Abide in Me, and I in you. As the branch cannot bear fruit of itself, unless it abides in the vine, neither can you, unless you abide in Me" (John 15:4, NKJV). God's part is to give us new motives, values, and attitudes. Our part is to stay connected to him and live out the new life he instills within.

When we invite God into our lives, we can have confidence that the Holy Spirit will work twenty-four hours a day to make us more loving. At times it may seem like we are going in reverse, but we must continue to trust his skill and transforming power. And if we let him, Jesus will not stop until we are spiritually mature, transparent, secure, loving disciples of the master.

DISCUSSION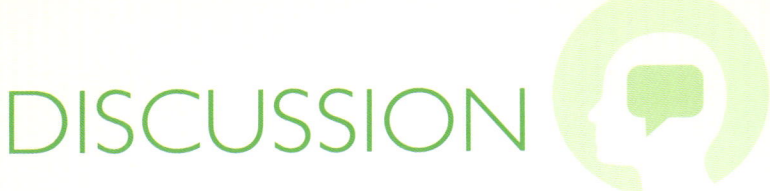

What do you imagine the man healed of leprosy talked about with his wife on his first night home?
....
....

Describe a time in your life when you felt isolated and alone. How did things turn around?
....
....

Share a time when you felt a healing touch of assurance and caring from someone.
....
....

What fears or insecurities can God's acceptance free us from?
....
....

If we are accepted by God "just as we are," what motivation is there to change?
....
....

What is our part in the process of spiritual growth? Describe.
....
....

If you were the surgeon in the imaginary hospital scenario in the lesson, how would you reassure the patient? How does that relate to the ways God reassures us?
....
....

In Ephesians 2:10, we are called God's "masterpiece." Why do you think Paul chose that word?
....
....

SHARING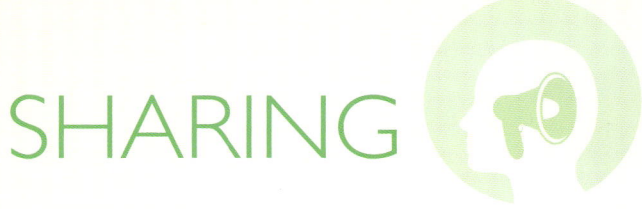

OPPORTUNITY #4:

- Pray as a group for God to open the way for you to share something from these lessons to help someone else.

- Keep your radar up each day for opportunities.

ABUNDANT LIVING THOUGHT

Jesus will make it as easy as possible for us to stay close to him and as difficult as possible for us to stray away.

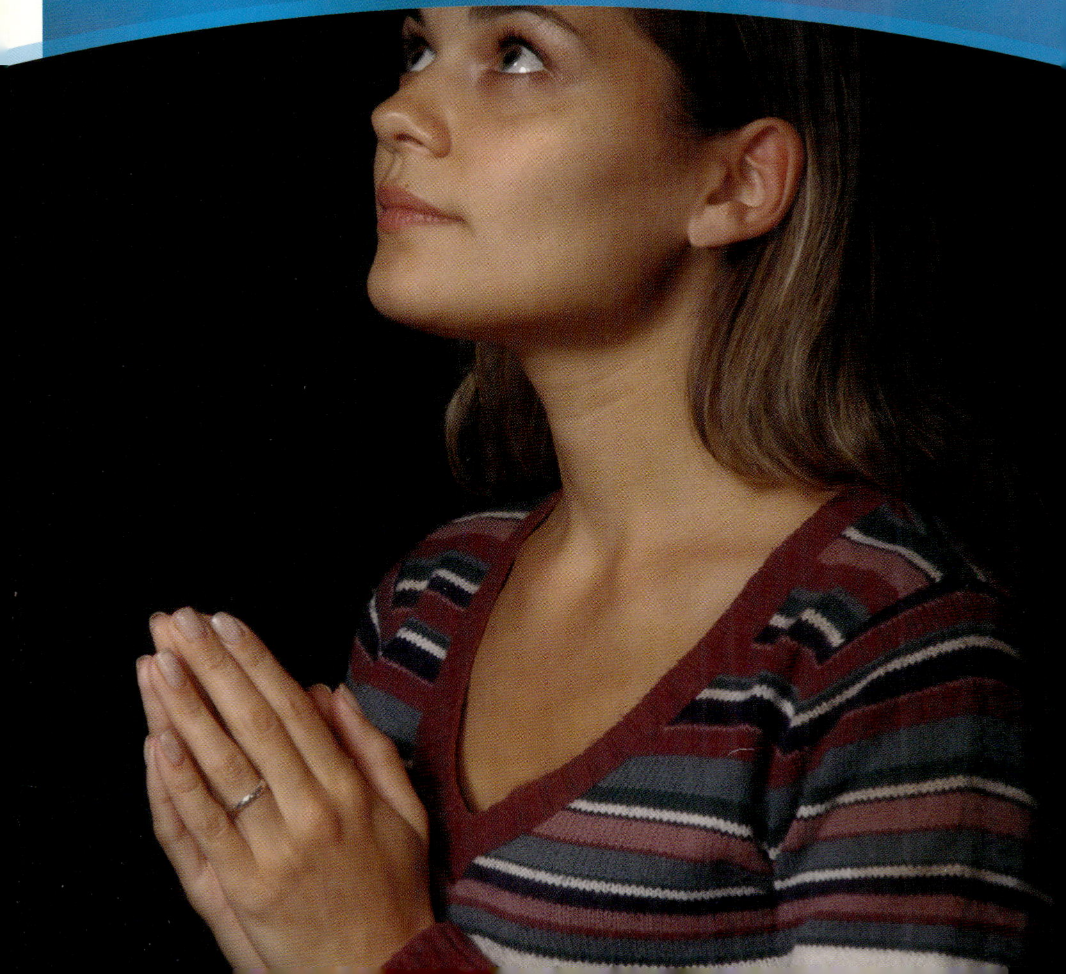

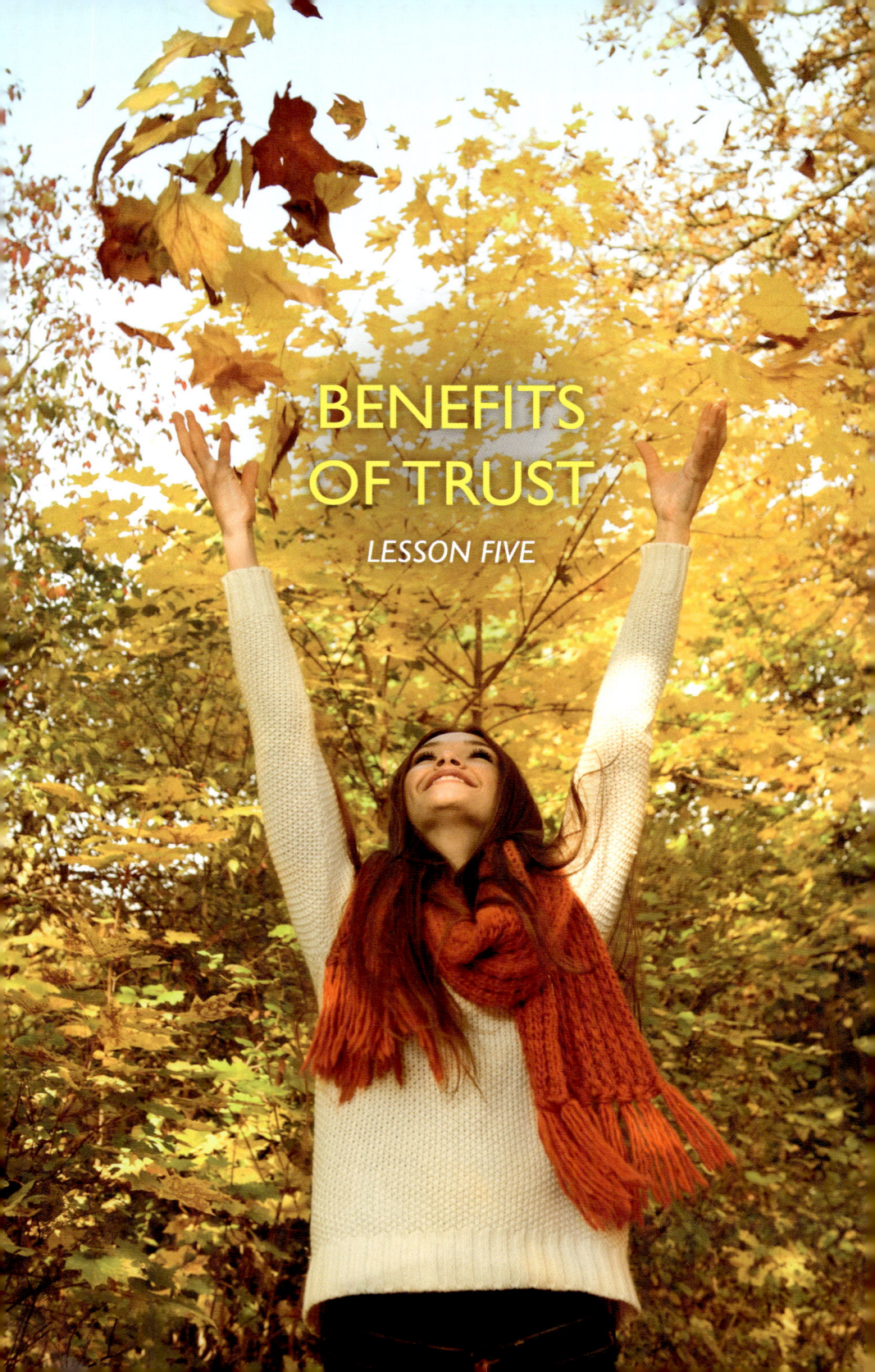

WARM UP

Feedback: In what ways did God open the door last week for you to share some part of the lesson with someone else?

....
....
....
....

Choose one or both questions to discuss (if in a group setting), or write out your answers on a separate sheet (for individual use):

1. **What do you wish your parents would have told you while you were still a kid?**[19]

....
....
....

2. **When you feel down, what helps renew your spirit?**[20]

....
....
....

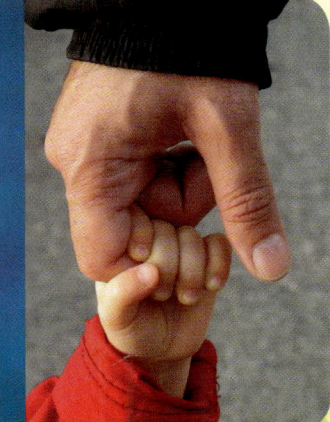

"When the core of our being is threatened, that's when we find out that trust is not something you have; trust is something you do moment-by-moment."

LINDA NORDYKE HAMBLETON

CREATION HEALTH | LIFE GUIDE #5

DISCOVERY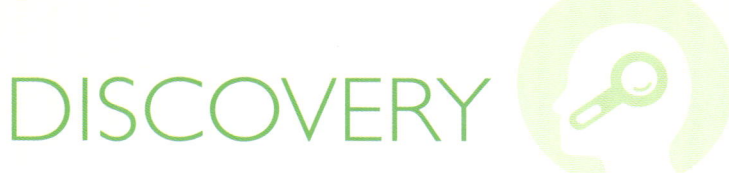

As we have seen so far, trust in God gives us access to salvation now and hope for the future. It is also the foundation of our ongoing love relationship with Christ. In this lesson we will explore some of the additional benefits such trust makes possible.

1. Trust In God and Holistic Health.

The spiritual dimension of life cannot be separated from the mental, emotional, and physical aspects of our being. All of these elements interact with one another and are intimately related. Based on that perspective, researchers have been exploring for some time how spirituality impacts our overall health. A number of exciting discoveries have emerged from their numerous investigations.

The following research included a focus on the health impact of an *individual's personal trust relationship with God*. We can only present here a small sampling:

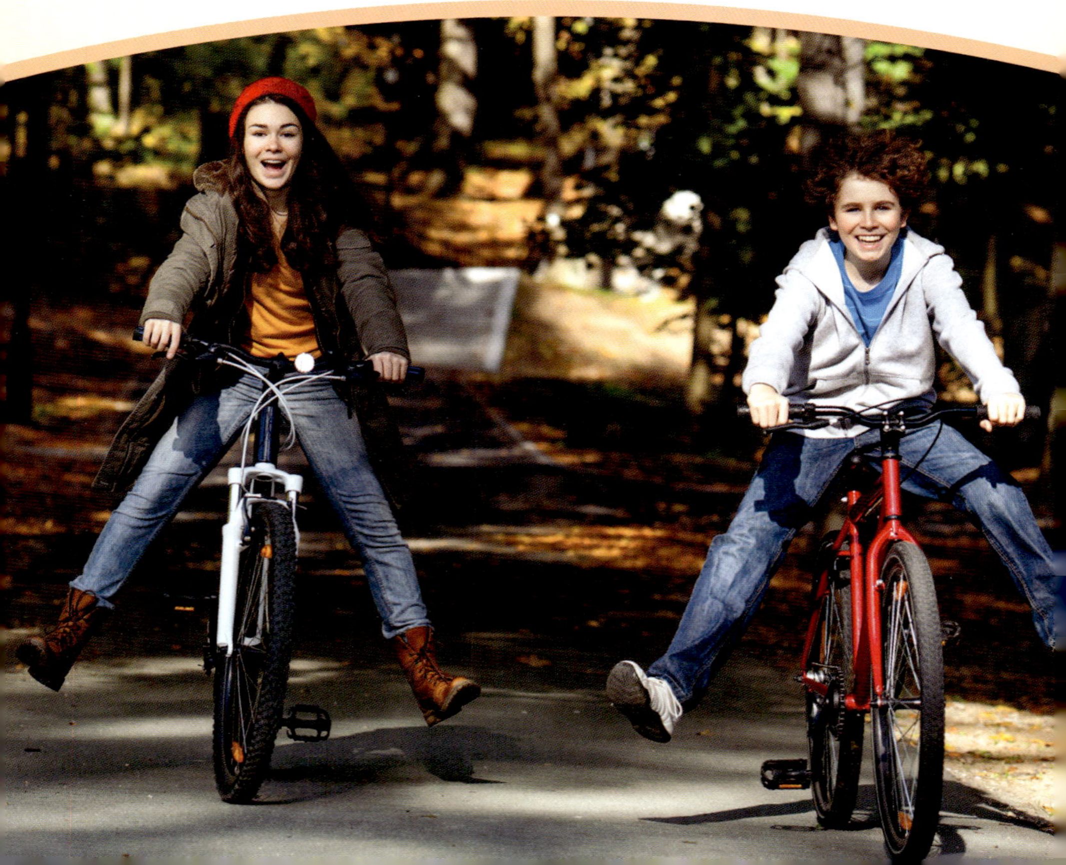

- **Better overall sense of well-being**
  The Americans' Changing Lives study of more than 1,500 adults revealed that people with a personal religious experience enjoyed greater life satisfaction.[21] The results of nearly eighty studies indicate a close association between religious involvement and an overall sense of well-being, including happiness, optimism, sense of meaning, and high morale.[22]

- **Lower blood pressure**
  Researchers from Duke University and the University of North Carolina studied over four hundred men in Evans County, Georgia. They were asked, "Quite aside from church going, how important in general would you say religion is to you?" The options were "very," "somewhat," and "not at all." Those that answered "very" enjoyed, on average, the lowest blood pressure readings.[23]

- **Protection against stress-related disorders**
  In a study at Harvard's behavioral medical clinic, eighty patients were given an assessment that measures twenty-five symptoms associated with stress disorders. The results indicated that personal spirituality had a very significant influence on reducing symptoms from stress and providing a protective effect over time.[24]

  Researcher Jeff Levin, PhD, gets at the root of why trust in God is such a powerful antidote to the corrosive effects of modern society. "Simple faith benefits health by leading to thoughts of hope, optimism, and positive expectation."[25]

- **Good mental health**
  In a study of 2,700 adults in New Haven, Connecticut, Dr. Ellen L. Idler, medical sociologist at Rutgers University, found a significant link between strong personal faith and good mental health.[26]

  Duke University psychiatrist and researcher, Dr. Harold G. Koenig, adds that religious faith "provides a mechanism by which attitudes can be changed and life circumstances reframed."[27]

- **Improved longevity**
  Several studies indicate that people who trust in God live longer, more fulfilling lives.[28] One research project, for example, showed that those who derived comfort from their faith were three times more likely to be living six months after open-heart surgery than those who had no such personal belief.[29]

2. Trust In God and Significance.

I remember well the day I played a tree in our elementary school play. Several students from grades five to eight were given actual words to say. Second graders like me were relegated to scenery. We were thought to be too forgetful and mumble-prone for speaking parts.

The trunk of my tree was made from a large cardboard box curved into a cylinder with a hole in the back for me to enter and a slit to see through in the front. It lacked realistic taper at the top, but no one seemed to mind. The limbs were cardboard cutouts, held on with duct tape. The entire outfit was then sprayed brown. To make sure the audience knew I was a living tree, the teacher stapled on several fake leaves made from green construction paper. Two handles on the inside gave my tree the magical ability to move.

Judging by my parents' excitement, you'd think I had landed the leading role in a Broadway play. On the big night, they came early to get seats down front. Other kids' parents did the same.

Those heady days of being cheered for simply being a tree in the background are long gone and I miss them dearly. Today, such a feeling of significance is hard to come by for the vast majority of us who occupy background positions in life. We can feel like simply one more unlauded face in the vast sea of humanity. There is no audience applauding our efforts as we faithfully carry out our daily routines. No curtain call for doing our part.

Trust in God dramatically changes that life-dulling scenario. You see, God celebrates each of us as if we were heroes. Whatever our chosen path in life, he sits in the front row and claps like crazy. God does not see crowds, only individuals. You are infinitely important to him, and he would have sent his Son Jesus Christ to die on a cross even if you were the only one who accepted him as savior. Put your name in the famous text, "God so loved [you], that he gave his only Son" (see John 3:16).

No matter how mundane your life may seem, no matter how insignificant you may feel, trust that you are of great significance to God. We matter so much to him that he even keeps updated on the number of hairs on our head! (Matt. 10:30).

3. Trust In God and Control.

We certainly have control over many aspects of our lives. Our level of fulfillment, satisfaction, happiness, and health are determined to a large degree by our own choices. Without question, the decisions we make as we journey through life impact our experience in a big way.

That personal sense of control is both calming and reassuring. But in many ways it is only an illusion. I could get hit by a drunk driver tomorrow night and be paralyzed. Lightning could hit my house and burn it to the ground. I could be diagnosed with cancer at my next annual physical and wind up in a fight for survival. I could get laid off and be unable to pay the mortgage.

We don't like to think about it, but we all know that our personal world is subject to forces far beyond our control. I don't suggest that we dwell on that reality throughout the day. But we can't keep those possibilities from undermining our peace to some degree.

That is where trust in God can make a huge difference. Bad stuff may happen, but that is not the end of the story. God gets involved in two important ways. First, he creates meaning from whatever may come our way. He takes the ups and downs of life and utilizes them to fit his purposes (see Rom. 8:28). Second, he is in charge of how we spend eternity.

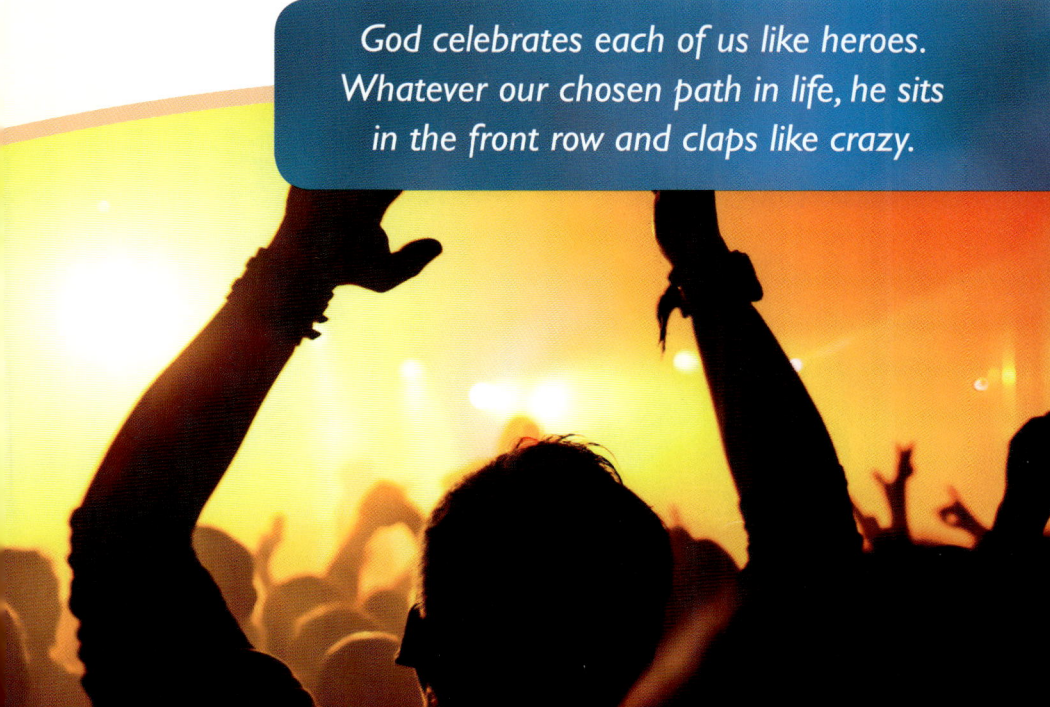

God celebrates each of us like heroes. Whatever our chosen path in life, he sits in the front row and claps like crazy.

I am reminded of the story of Corrie ten Boom, who was placed in a Nazi concentration camp during World War II because she provided a hiding place for Jews. Her father and sister were also arrested and died before the camps were liberated by the Allies. Many years later, in her eighties, she appeared in a documentary and recounted those terrible days.

The camera zooms in on Corrie as she works on some needlepoint in her lap. She eventually concludes her story by holding up the backside of the needlepoint with its tangle of criss-crossed threads going this way and that in no apparent order. She comments, "This is the side of our lives that we see." She then turns the needlepoint over, showing a beautiful pattern that spells out the words, "God is love." Corrie smiles and says, "This is the side of our lives that God sees."[30]

God does not cause hard times, but he can incorporate any dark threads into the beautiful tapestry of our lives. He also controls our ultimate destiny. Whatever life sends our way, God will have the final word.

> *God does not cause hard times, but he can incorporate any dark threads into the beautiful tapestry of our lives.*

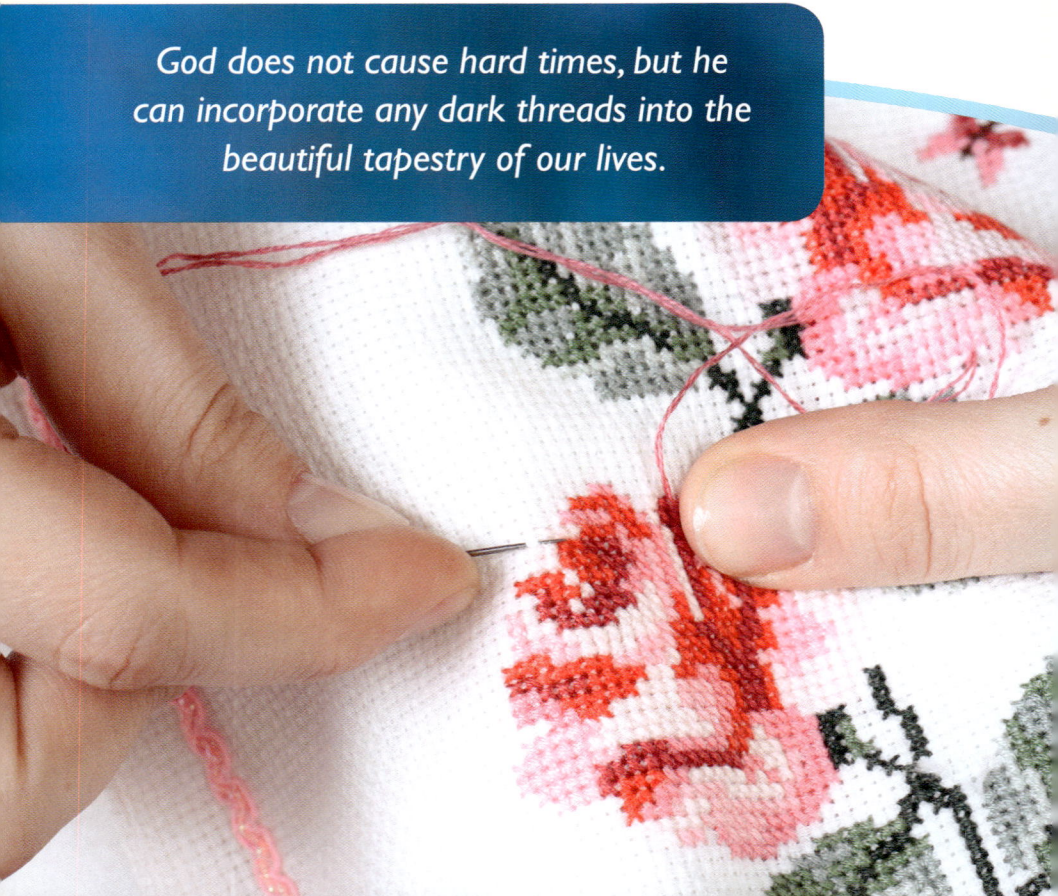

4. Trust In God and Following Your Heart.

T-ball is baseball for little kids. Rather than someone pitching the ball, it sits on a thin pole in front of them and they simply attempt to whack it as far as they can from there. Tracy loved to play but rarely connected bat with ball. She had coke-bottle glasses, hearing aids in each ear, and had to pull one leg after her when she ran.

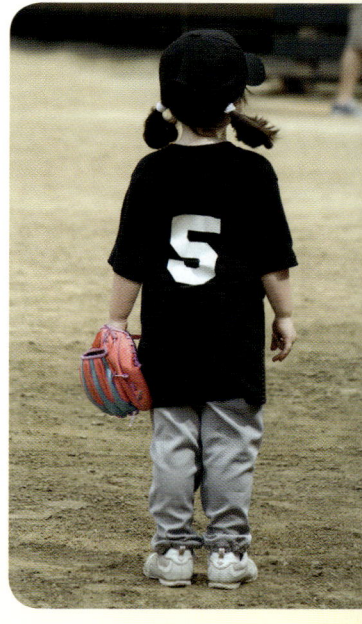

During the final game of the season, against all odds, Tracy somehow creamed the ball. It shot straight up the middle through the legs of multiple players into the far reaches of the outfield. Tracy stood on home plate transfixed. Everyone yelled, "Run, run!" With parents screaming, the young girl loped down to first, then on to second, slowly rounded third, and headed home while several kids tracked down the distant ball.

And then it happened. During the pandemonium, a tired, twelve-year-old dog lumbered close to the baseline, wagging its tail at all the excitement. Tracy stopped, thirty feet from her first ever home run. People urged her to continue. Instead, she turned, smiled, followed her heart, and went for the dog.[31] Two roads diverged at that moment in Tracy's life, the road of expectations and the road of love. Tracy chose love.

When we sign on with Jesus, he invites us to follow Tracy's example and listen to our hearts. Jesus never allowed others' expectations to dictate his life, and he longs for us to bring some of that same sense of adventure and freedom into our own lives.

Jesus is not calling us to be reckless or irresponsible, but he is calling us to trust his example and stop allowing ourselves to be dictated to by the crowd. Dare to rekindle some long-neglected vision, some postponed yearning, then follow God's lead by giving yourself permission to color outside the lines. Don't simply do the predictable action on every occasion. Make time for your dream. Give it priority. It may be a goal, a project, a hobby, or a relationship. Invite Jesus to help shape and modify that dream to produce the best possible outcome and trust that he will.

5. Trust In God and Human Suffering.

For centuries people have posed the question, "Why does God allow so much suffering in the world?" Books have been written attempting to answer that daunting question, so we cannot address it fully here. But I do want to at least steer readers away from the kind of fruitless, spirit-sapping search for answers that I engaged in for years. I have concluded that there are no answers to that question this side of eternity.

In reality, we should be asking a very different question, "How do we integrate a lack of answers into our Christian experience?" Put another way, "How do we live with mystery?"

God gave us an important clue in his dialogue with Job in the Old Testament. Job had endured horrible losses, and even though he hung in there spiritually, he was deeply troubled by the fact that God allowed it to happen.

God's response is to remind Job of his infinite power and transcendence:

> *Where were you when I created the earth?*
> *Who came up with the blueprints and measurements?*
> *Do you know where Light comes from*
> *and where Darkness lives*
> *Can you get the attention of the clouds,*
> *and commission a shower of rain?*
> *Can you take charge of the lightning bolts*
> *and have them report to you for orders?*
> *(Job 38: 4, 5, 19, 34–35, MSG).*

Such a response may seem indirect, but it is actually very helpful. God is reminding us that he is infinitely powerful and wise. He operates in a realm that is far beyond our ability to fully comprehend now. It is this very transcendence that opens the door for there to be satisfying answers that my little brain cannot understand in this sinful world.

I already trust God for the answers to other huge mysteries such as, "How can God have no beginning?" and "How can the vast universe have no end?" The path forward for me in dealing with the harsh reality of human suffering is to trust him for that mystery as well. I trust that, as the infinite one, he will one day provide powerful answers that I cannot even begin to imagine now. And I trust that when sin is finally vanquished, we will experience what the prophet saw in a vision, "God will wipe away every tear from their eyes; there shall be no more death, nor sorrow, nor crying. There shall be no more pain, for the former things have passed away" (Rev. 21:4, NKJV).

> God will wipe away every tear from their eyes.

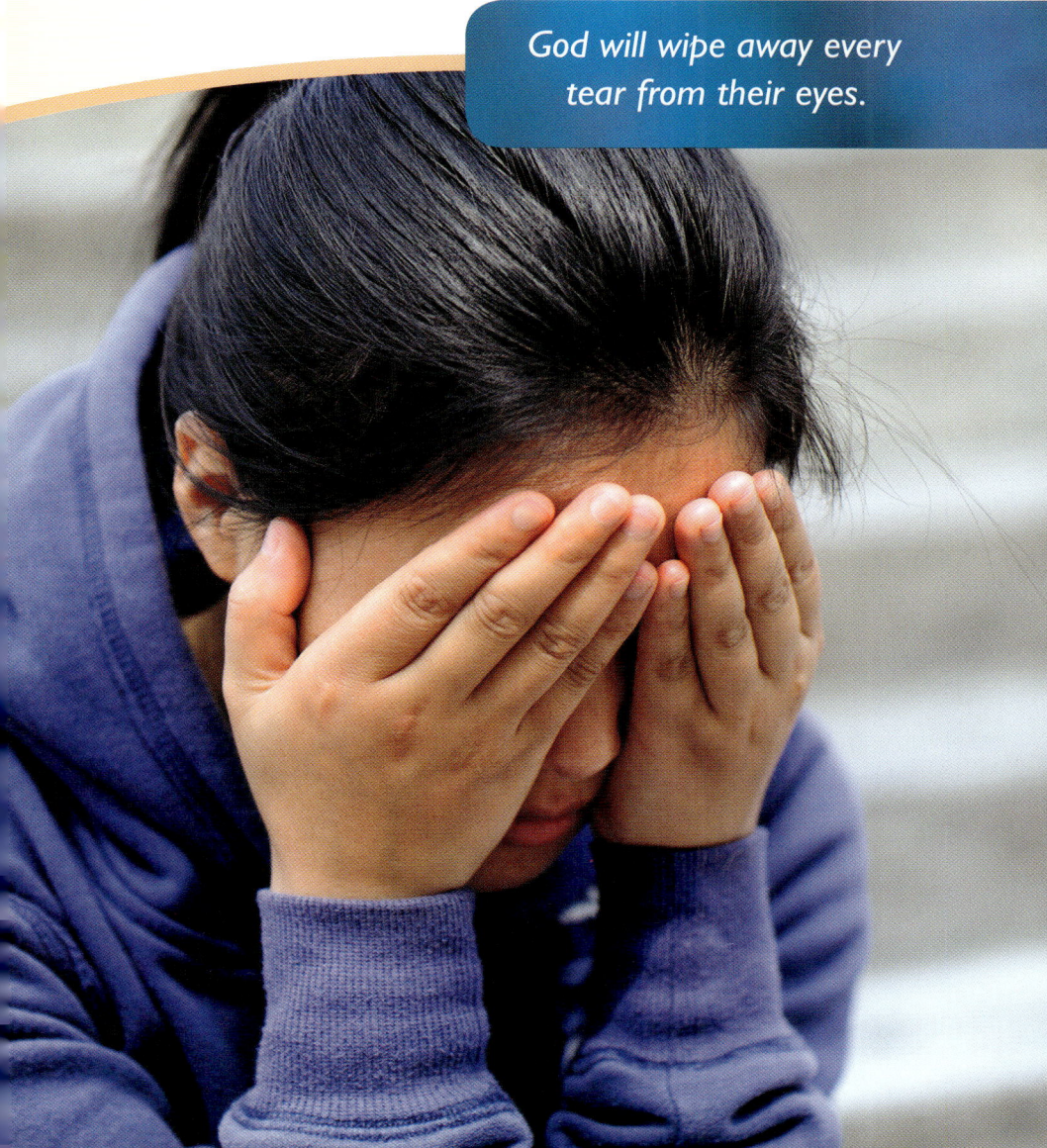

DISCUSSION

Are there any holistic health benefits from trusting God that you have experienced personally? Describe.

....
....

What does the term "life satisfaction" mean to you?

....
....

Describe some ways that trust in God helps you emotionally.

....
....

How would you define a feeling of significance? Why is it so essential?

....
....

How important is "being in control" to you? Why are some people "control freaks"?

....
....

What are you particularly trusting God for now?

....
....

What does it mean to allow God to be in charge of our life? How does he take charge?

....
....

Describe a time when you ignored the expectations of others and "followed your heart."

....
....

SHARING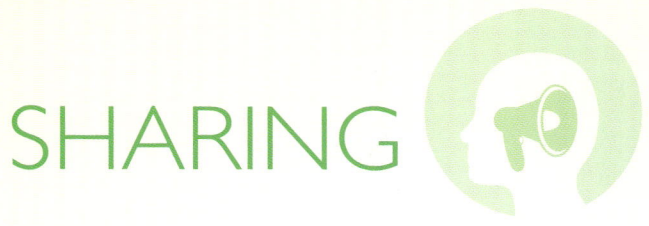

OPPORTUNITY #5:

- Pray as a group for God to open the way for you to share something from these lessons to help someone else.

- Keep your radar up each day for opportunities.

ABUNDANT LIVING THOUGHT

No matter how mundane your life may seem, no matter how insignificant you may feel, trust that you are of great significance to God.

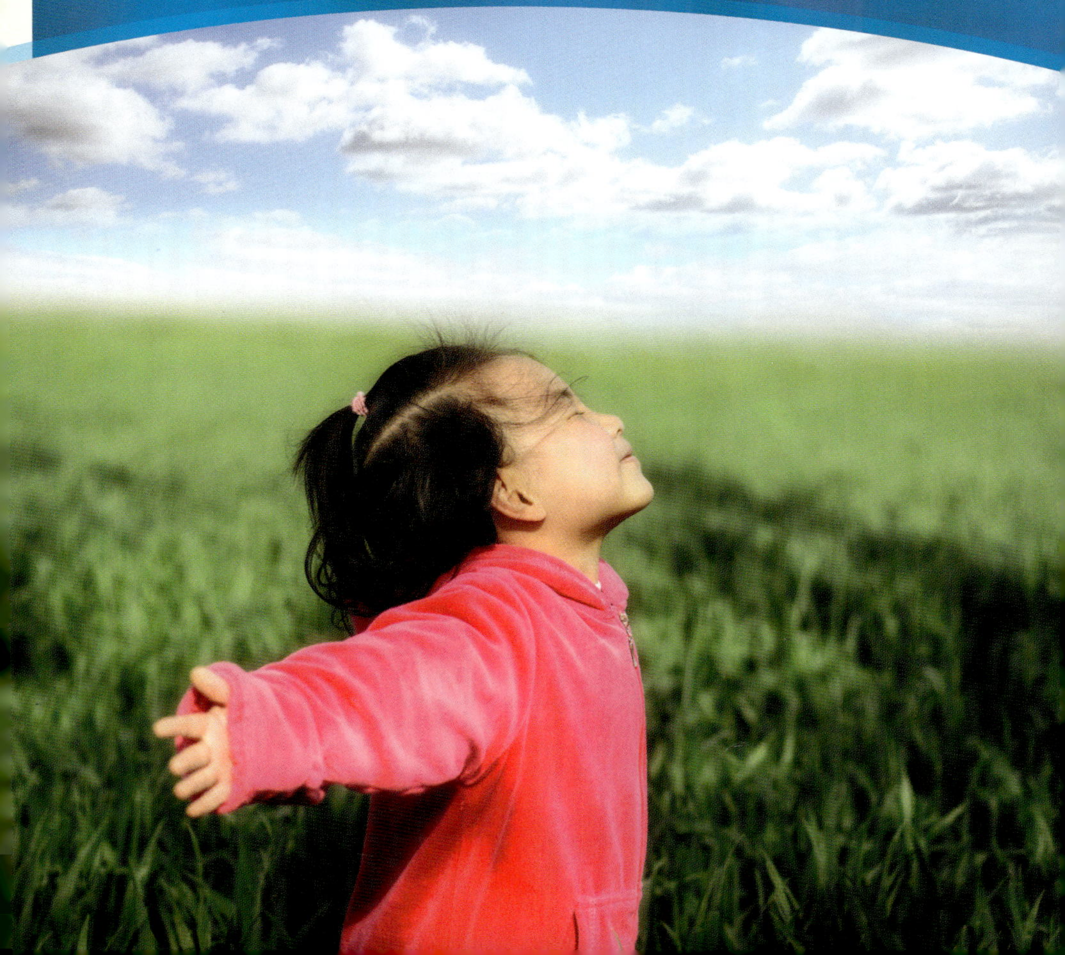

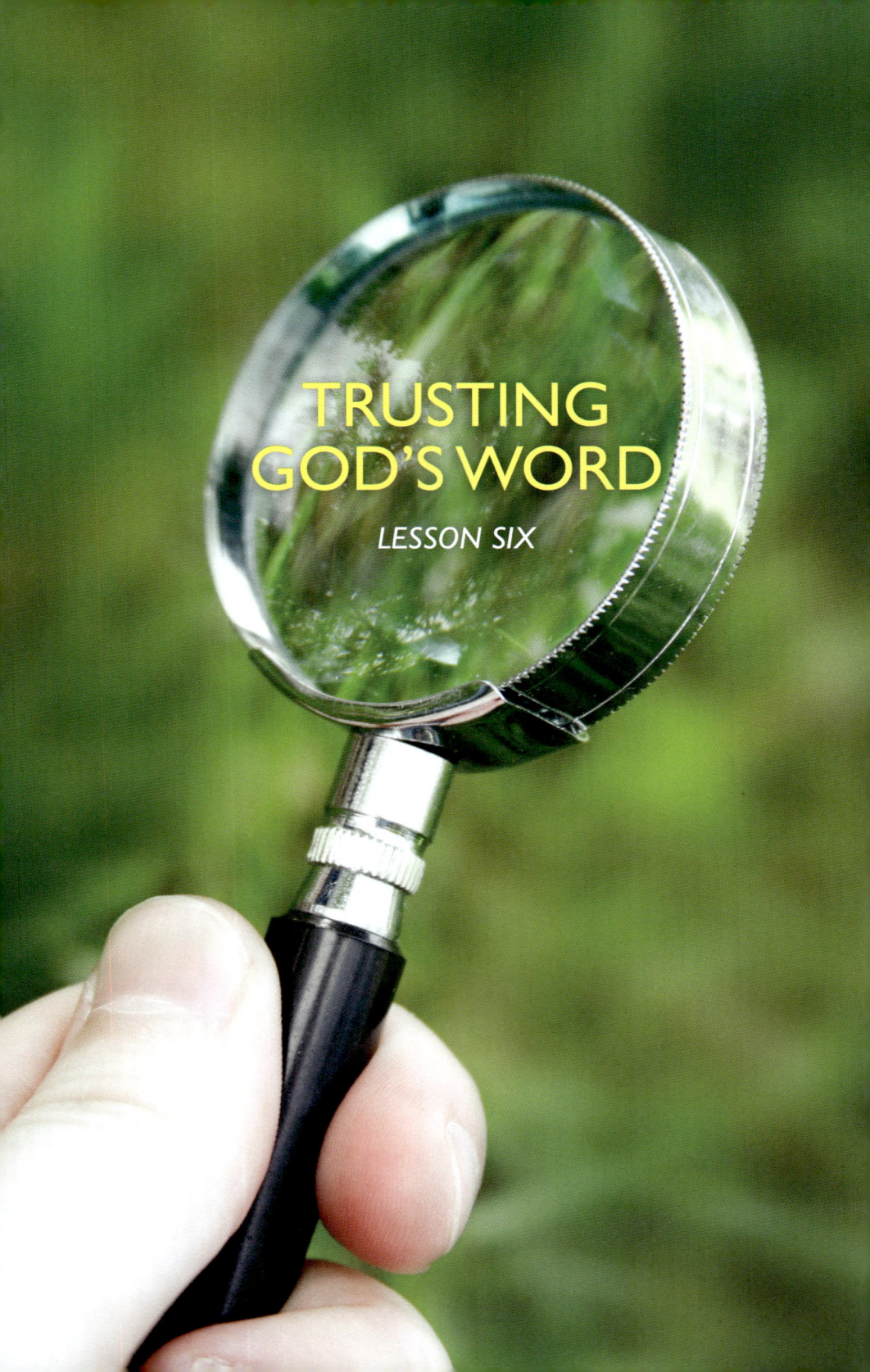

WARM UP

Feedback: In what ways did God open the door last week for you to share some part of the lessons with someone else?

....
....
....
....

Choose one or both questions to discuss (if in a group setting), or write out your answers on a separate sheet (for individual use):

1. **Generally speaking, what is the best way for two people to resolve a conflict?**[32]

....
....
....

2. **Describe one of your most satisfying experiences in school.**

....
....
....

> *The truth is, you have captured God's heart and won his affection.*
>
> **TODD CHOBOTAR**

DISCOVERY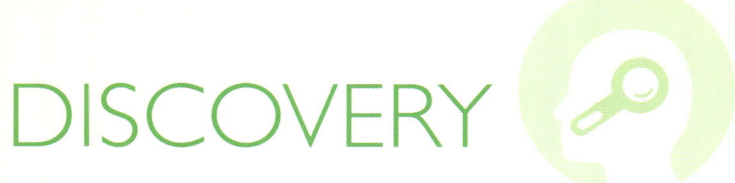

The prank eventually became a part of office legend.

The office building interior desperately needed updating and, as office manager, my boss supervised the project. For some reason he took a special interest in replacing the carpet – canvassing the staff about color, visiting stores, getting advice over the phone, reading articles. He brought back so many samples that his office looked like an outlet.

After weeks of research, the momentous decision was finally made – solid mauve. To me it was simply purple, but what did I know?

Out with the old and in with the new. The carpet looked great and my boss was more than pleased. For days, every visitor got the back story and a tour. "Yah, I looked at all kinds of weaves, colors, grades. Not an easy task, I'll tell you that. But it all paid off. Yes sir, really takes the office to a whole new level, don't you think?"

Besides being a top grade carpet picker-outer, my boss was also a professional prankster. Being two-time targets, the other associate and I saw a golden opportunity to balance the scales. We copied the letterhead from the carpet company's copious correspondence with our department and addressed a bogus letter from them to our boss. It read:

> We have just received an urgent notification from the Centers for Disease Control in Atlanta, GA. We regret to inform you that the carpet we recently installed at your location contains new dyes that can cause dangerous flu-like symptoms. The CDC has issued a complete recall and that color will no longer be available. Our installers will be contacting you for carpet removal in the next few days.

We sent it regular mail to give it an air of credibility, then waited. Sure enough, the very next day you could hear the howls all the way down the hall. "What on earth? I can't believe it! After all that work! This is the stupidest thing I've ever heard!"

Mercifully, we only let him fume for a few minutes before telling him the truth. Good-natured smiles and chuckles all around. He admired our ingenuity.

The letter illustrates the need for healthy caution when it comes to some kinds of communication. Not all information is accurate. Not all documents can be trusted. The issue of credibility is particularly vital when the communication is about highly significant matters. The more important the contents, the more important trust becomes.

Such is the case with Scripture. The Scriptures are the foundation of our understanding of God, and it is essential for us to have confidence in their veracity. We need to know that what the Bible says accurately reflects the thinking of its author *because trust in God comes through trust in the Bible.*

The authenticity of Scripture came under unusually sharp attack during the first half of the twentieth century. Those attacks were not without their effect, subtly eroding many people's confidence, even at the local church level. That impact has lingered. Two of the main criticisms could be summarized as follows:

1. **Document transmission** – how can documents that were repeatedly copied by hand from generation to generation possibly be accurate?

2. **Historical records** – how can the names of people and places in the Bible be correct if they don't show up anywhere in ancient, non-biblical history or literature?

Since the time these two challenges were originally put forth, much has changed. Today we are able to provide some remarkable answers, and believers' confidence in Scripture has been dramatically affirmed. We only have space in this lesson to highlight a few of the most significant developments.

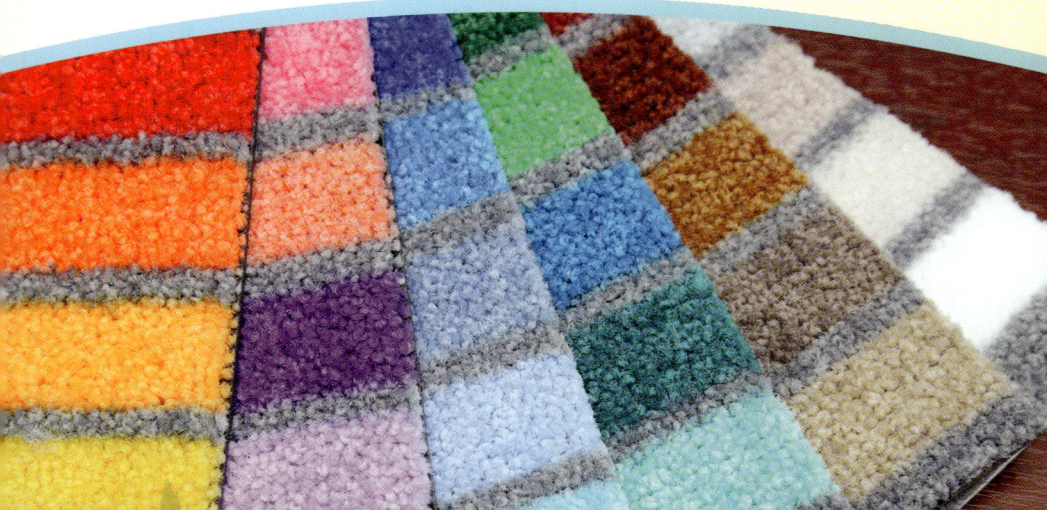

DOCUMENT TRANSMISSION

It is true that we have none of the original manuscripts from any of the Bible writers. Those parchments deteriorated long, long ago, from use, age, and climate. What we do have are copies. Actually, we have copies of copies of copies, etc., that were made down through the centuries. Doubts regarding the accuracy of those handmade copies were answered in dramatic fashion in the year 1947.

During that year, in the area of the Middle East called Khirbet Qumran, on the shores of the Dead Sea, a shepherd boy roamed the hills looking for his lost sheep.[33] At some point he threw a rock into a cave located high up on a cliff. Instead of hearing the familiar sound of rock on rock, he heard what seemed very much like the cracking of pottery. Curiosity aroused, the young Bedouin climbed up to investigate. As his eyes adjusted to the semi-darkness, he saw, to his amazement, several large clay jars containing old leather scrolls carefully wrapped in linen.[34]

More interested in money for food than keeping ancient scrolls, the shepherd lad grabbed an armful of history and headed off to find an antiques buyer in Jerusalem. Those were days of terrible turmoil within Israel leading up to the Arab-Israeli War, and the scrolls could very easily have been bartered away into oblivion.[35] Instead, they eventually wound up in safe, capable hands at St. Mark's Monastery in Old Jerusalem and Hebrew University.[36]

Excitement over the scrolls led to official examination of the entire cave area. More caves were discovered with thousands of manuscript fragments and hundreds more scrolls. After years of painstaking reconstruction, researchers found portions of every book of the Old Testament except Esther, plus a complete copy of the book of Isaiah.[37]

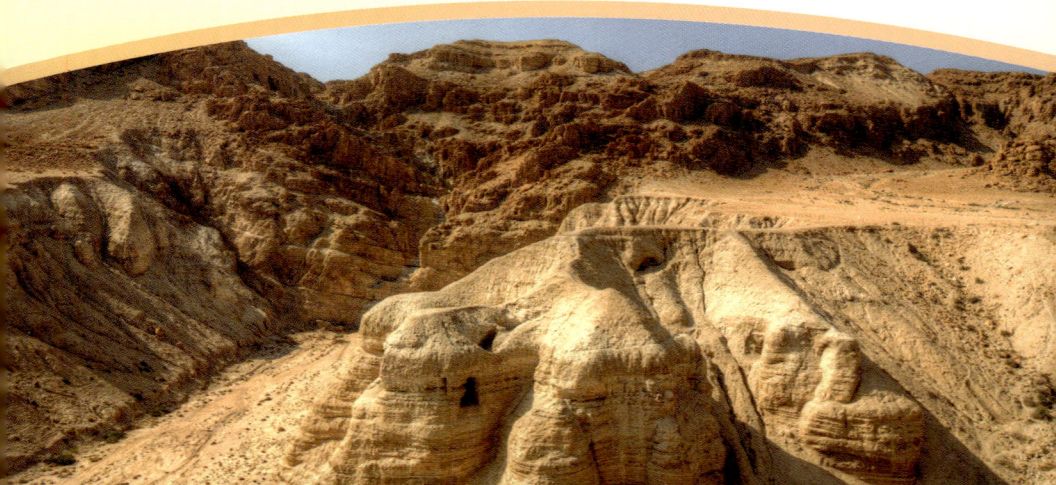

For many years the oldest Hebrew manuscripts of the Old Testament that we had were from around 900 AD forward.[38] When the Dead Sea scrolls were finally dated, they turned out to have come from approximately one to two hundred years before Christ! That means that the scrolls take us an astonishing 1,000 years further back in time, and the pressing question was how they compared to the much newer manuscripts? One thousand years is a very long time, and Christians around the globe held their collective breath to see the results of a careful comparison. Had significant errors crept in from the copiers' hands?

Bible researchers were hopeful because they knew that ancient copyists were trained specialists who worked in a supervised environment where strict rules and guidelines were followed. All of these individuals were also raised to have a deep, personal reverence for Scripture.

So what was the result from comparing the manuscripts from around 900 AD to the Dead Sea scrolls from 100–200 BC? Bottom line was that the copyists during that time did a remarkable job. Professor Eugene Ulrich summarizes the conclusion of biblical scholars when he writes, "The scrolls have shown that our traditional Bible has been amazingly accurately preserved."[39] After studying the scrolls of Qumran, Dr. Will Varner, professor of Old Testament in Israel, states, "We can have confidence that our Old Testament Scriptures faithfully represent the words given to Moses, David, and the prophets."[40] Gerhard Pfandl, PhD, adds, "No other ancient writings comparable to the Old Testament have been transmitted so accurately."[41]

The Dead Sea Scrolls provide spine-tingling proof that the Old Testament Scriptures we hold in our hands today can indeed be trusted.

We can also have strong confidence that the New Testament was faithfully transmitted as well. Edward Glenny declares, "God has given us 5,656 manuscripts containing all or parts of the Greek NT. It is the most remarkably preserved book in the ancient world. Not only do we have a great number of manuscripts but they are very close in time to the originals they represent."[42] F.F. Bruce observes, "There is no body of ancient literature in the world which enjoys such a wealth of good textual attestation as the New Testament."[43]

HISTORICAL RECORDS

There are many towns, cities, people groups, and events named in Scripture that could not be found in any secular literature from the past. "Surely these supposed facts must be myths," the critics claimed, "or else we'd find them mentioned elsewhere." The issue is important because if the Bible can be proven to be inaccurate regarding historical facts, what else could it be inaccurate about?

Archaeology has come to the rescue in incredible ways, unearthing evidence that consistently corroborates the biblical account. Joseph Free observes, "In addition to illuminating the Bible, archaeology has confirmed countless passages which have been rejected by critics as unhistorical or contradictory to known facts."[44] Some people groups and places in Scripture remain unverified still, but enough have been confirmed to give us plenty of reason to trust.

There are numerous stories of how archaeology has established the biblical account. We only have space for a few examples:

- Secular historians taught that the biblical account of a people called the Hittites was inaccurate and that Belshazzar, the king of the Chaldeans who Daniel wrote about, never existed. Archaeologists have now vindicated the accuracy of Scripture in both cases.[45]

- For many years critics said that King David in the Old Testament was a myth because he was never mentioned in any secular history. On July 21, 1993, that picture changed dramatically, when Avraham Biran of Hebrew Union College and his team of Israeli archaeologists were excavating the ruins of the ancient city of Dan. Gila Cook discovered a flattened basalt stone that contained an inscription. Dated from the ninth century BC, it commemorated a military victory over King David and the House of David. It was, to say the least, a momentous confirmation of the biblical account.[46]

- Critics argued that Luke's account of the census taken at the time of Jesus' birth was pure fiction. However, all of the facts mentioned in the gospel – the census itself, the fact that Quirinius was governor of Syria, and the requirement that everyone return to their ancestral home – have now been confirmed by non-biblical sources (see Luke 2:1–2). Noted historian and archaeologist, Sir William Ramsey, concludes, "Luke is a historian of the first rank."[47]

- The gospel of John mentions a pool called Bethesda just inside an entrance to the city of Jerusalem at the Sheep Gate. He specifies that it had five porches (John 5:2, NKJV). The problem was that no such pool design had ever been mentioned in any ancient source. Critics chalked it up to John's imagination. Modern archaeologists decided to dig precisely where John indicated. They soon came upon a pool from that time period with exactly five porticoes, just as the gospel described it.[48]

- In 1961, Italian archaeologists uncovered a special two-foot by three-foot limestone block during their excavations of an ancient Roman amphitheatre located in the ruins of the seaside city of Caesarea Maritima. It contained an inscription that included the phrase, "Pontius Pilate, Prefect of Judea." The stone was apparently moved from its original location where it served to commemorate a temple Pilate built for the worship of Tiberias Caesar, the Roman emperor during Pilate's term of office in Judea. Although Josephus and Philo mention Pilate in their writings, the "Pilate Stone" provides invaluable contemporary confirmation of both his title and the territory over which he ruled. It is the only known occurrence of the ruler's name in an inscription.[49]

The Dead Sea Scrolls and the archaeologist's spade serve as powerful reminders that the God who inspired the Scriptures has wonderfully preserved them down through time. Today we can fully trust that they are, in fact, a true and reliable record of divine history and teaching.

Archaeology has come to the rescue in incredible ways, unearthing evidence that consistently corroborates the biblical account.

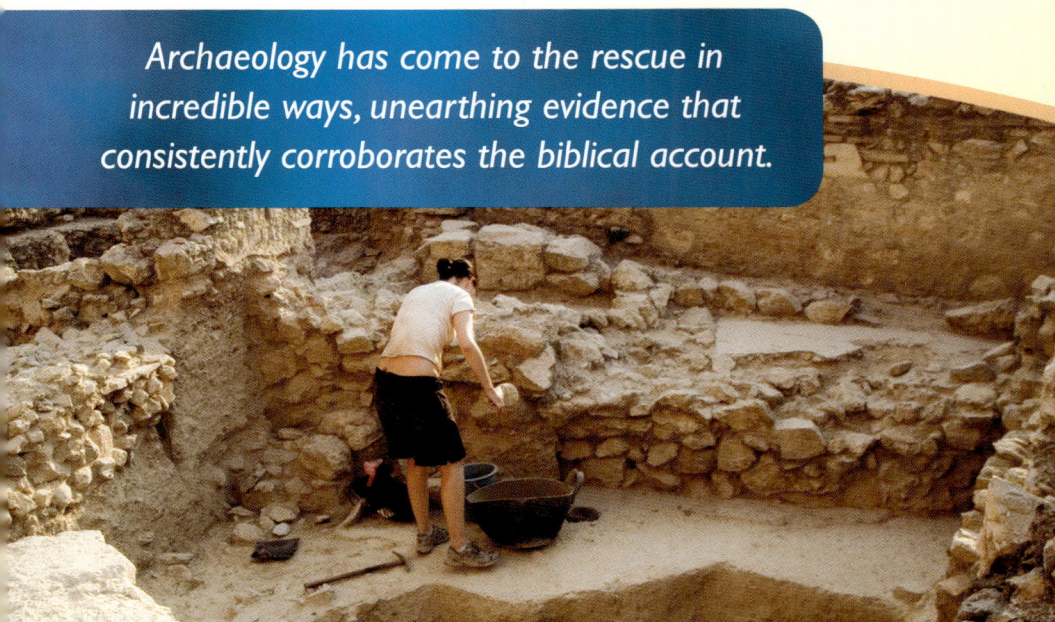

DISCUSSION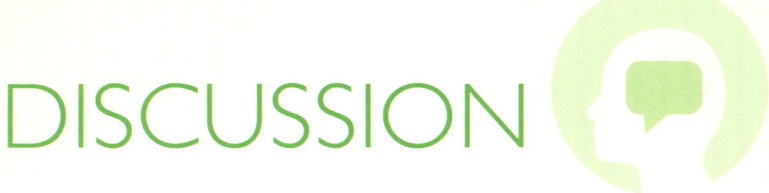

Describe a prank you pulled off successfully or one where you were the victim.
....
....

What caused ancient copyists to have such deep reverence for Scripture? Why has so much of that attitude been lost today?
....
....

What aspect of the story of the Dead Sea Scrolls do you find most interesting? Why?
....
....

If you were in charge of several copyists two thousand years ago, what rules or procedures would you put in place to make sure they did accurate work?
....
....

How does the accuracy of copying Scripture impact your trust in God?
....
....

How does the archaeological confirmation of Bible history help your confidence in Scripture?
....
....

How is your belief in historical figures such as Caesar or Shakespeare similar to or different from your belief in Bible characters?
....
....

How have you seen God's Word come alive in your own life recently?
....
....

SHARING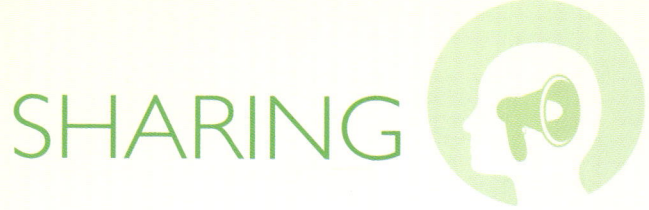

OPPORTUNITY #6:

- Pray as a group for God to open the way for you to share something from these lessons to help someone else.

- Keep your radar up each day for opportunities.

ABUNDANT LIVING THOUGHT

The Dead Sea Scrolls provide spine-tingling proof that the Old Testament Scriptures we hold in our hands today can indeed be trusted.

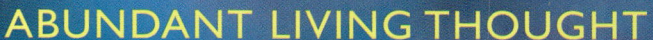

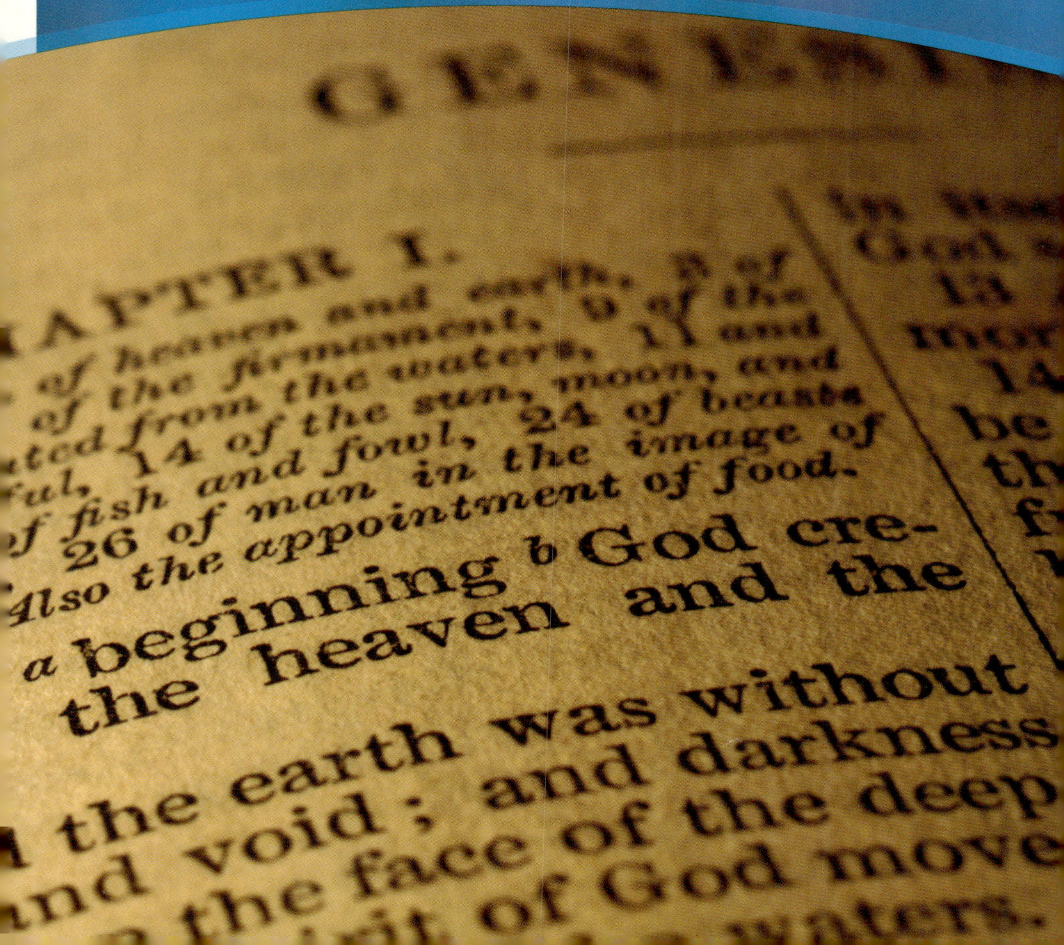

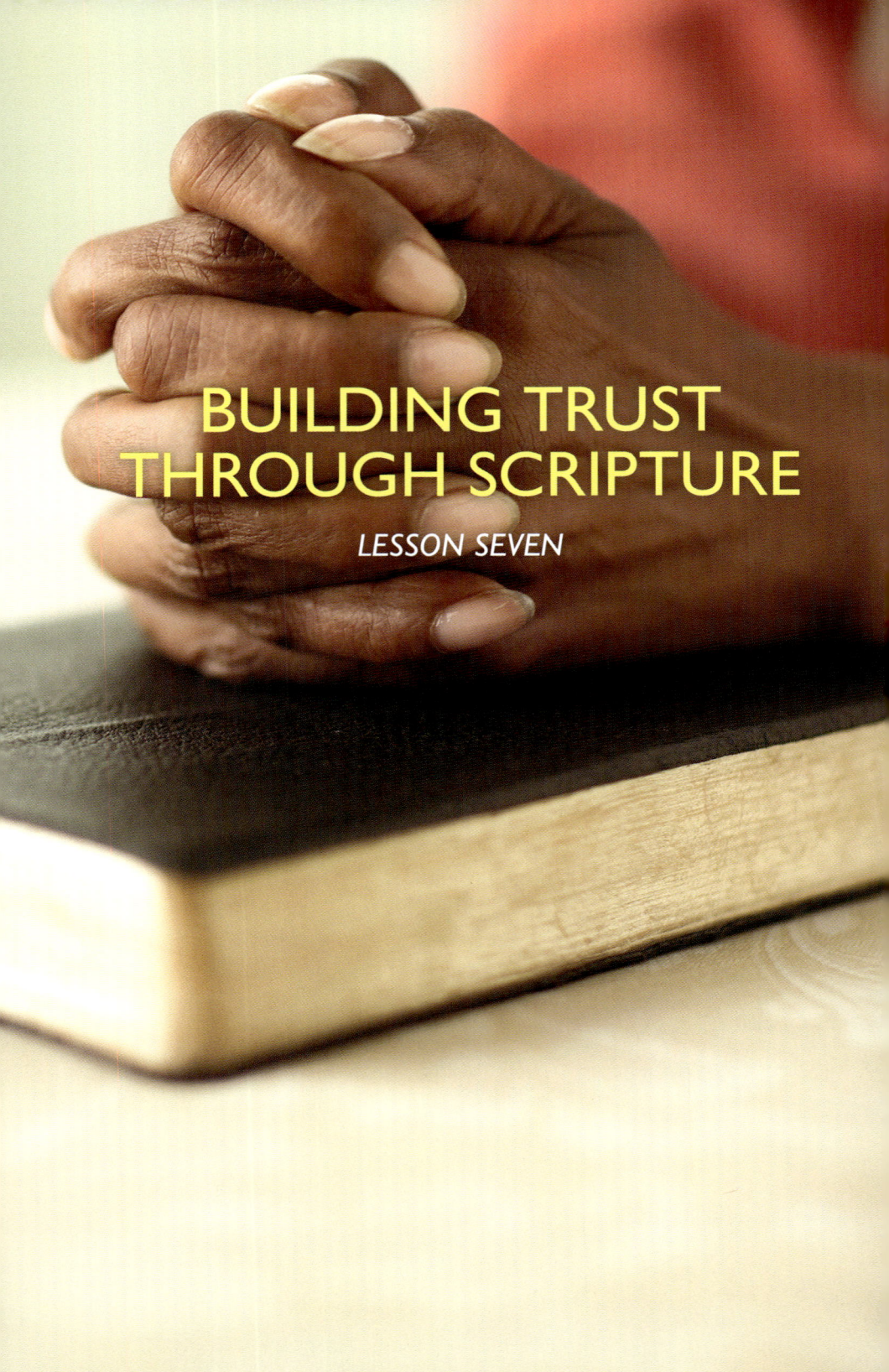

BUILDING TRUST THROUGH SCRIPTURE

LESSON SEVEN

WARM UP

Feedback: In what ways did God open the door last week for you to share some part of the lessons with someone else?

....
....
....
....

Choose one or both questions to discuss (if in a group setting), or write out your answers on a separate sheet (for individual use):

1. **Would you rather meet someone for the first time who was an interesting talker or a great listener? Why?**

....
....
....

2. **Where do you dream of taking a vacation? Why would you choose this location?**[50]

....
....
....

> *After spending time alone with God, we find that he injects into our bodies energy, power, and strength.*
>
> **CHARLES STANLEY**

DISCOVERY

I took an online course about four years ago that made me want to tear my little bit of remaining hair out. The class was intended for individuals who had a special interest in designing online instruction. According to the course description, it was supposed to focus on how to remove roadblocks from the learning process. By roadblocks it meant anything that hindered the student from understanding the material and applying it in a useful way. I was psyched.

The first assignment, however, already spelled trouble. We were supposed to download the latest version of a program from a website and use it to complete a lengthy project. I went to the website and had to create a login. After entering a carefully considered username and password, a little memo popped up that said, essentially, "What you just did is completely unacceptable!"

I paused, looked around the page for any hints about what I should do differently. No clues. Several more attempts met with increasingly fervent rejections. I checked the course chat room but saw no mention of any login problems. Too embarrassed to ask fellow students, I e-mailed the teacher as a last resort. He sent me a course-related username that "everyone was supposed to be using."

> *The Bible is the instruction manual on what trust in God is all about.*

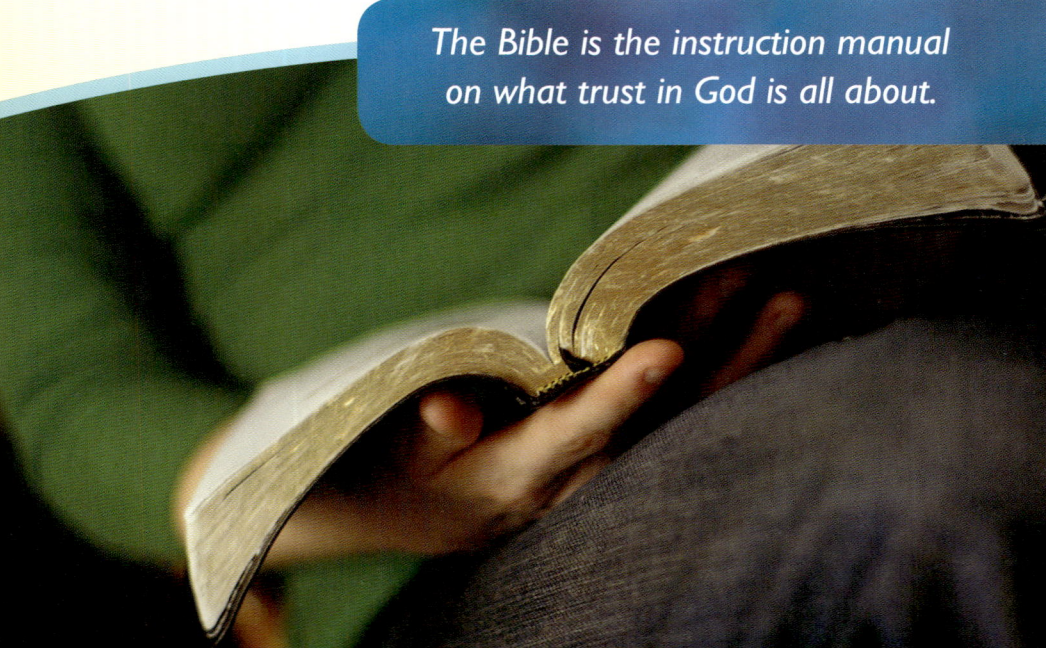

Eventually the program downloaded successfully, but now I had no idea how to use it. No notes were provided. No online manual. I dithered around with mounting frustration. Click here. Click there. I entered the chat room again and everyone else seemed to be using the program like an old pro. I felt like a bumbling outsider.

Beyond that, the teacher kept using three-letter abbreviations in his communications. For example, "As you know, the CBR is a great resource." Or, "Each student should consult the NRZ and the JQR to find articles that relate to the assignment." Bottom line, the course on eliminating roadblocks to learning was loaded with roadblocks! I dropped it after four weeks.

I think the fundamental problem was that the course assumed a level of understanding and orientation that I didn't have. I had somehow inadvertently wandered into a class that was on level 5 when I was still on level 1, or less. They had some vital inside information without which I floundered.

Many times people can feel the same way when it comes to studying the Bible. We hear a preacher or some other religious leader expound about how meaningful the Scriptures are for them. How they love delving into the Bible and how fulfilling they find it. The problem is that regular Christians are seldom taught how to study the Bible so it can be just as meaningful and fulfilling for them. There is an assumption that people know how to study the Bible, but that is too often simply not the case. The course entitled, "Personal Bible Study," can be full of roadblocks just like my online class.

All of this takes on particular importance when it comes to trusting God because *the Bible is the instruction manual on what trust in God is all about.* It is the primary source. And if it is unclear how to study the Scriptures in an effective way, our trust in him will suffer.

The Bible teaches us about trust in God in a variety of ways. We see how numerous individuals learned to trust him through all the ups and downs of their spiritual journeys and how failure to trust can cause heartache and confusion. We read how different authors explain the multi-faceted dimensions of trust. Most importantly, we learn about God himself, and the more we know him, the more we'll trust him.

Two Scripture verses are particularly relevant here. The general public in the apostle Paul's day didn't have written copies of the Old Testament. They learned from what they heard at the temple. Paul therefore writes, "So then faith [trust] comes by hearing, and hearing by the word of God" (Rom. 10:17, NKJV). He later commended Timothy for his understanding of Scripture, highlighting the connection between Bible study and faith. "From childhood you have known the Holy Scriptures, which are able to make you wise for salvation through faith which is in Christ Jesus" (2 Tim 3:15, NKJV).

In this lesson we will look at some key approaches to understanding the Bible. We will list strategies for exploring Scripture that many have found beneficial. As you read through this material, select what fits your needs best.

It can be helpful to distinguish between "Bible reading" and "Bible study."[51] *Reading* is for daily time with God, lasting between ten to thirty minutes. It is most often done in the morning to get you oriented for the day. *Study*, on the other hand, is a more lengthy examination of Scripture, from one to two hours using a variety of study aids and books to help you delve more deeply into portions of the Bible. That will typically occur less often than your daily reading, but at least once a week.

There are, of course, a variety of ways that reading and study can be designed and scheduled. The important point here is to make a distinction between the two. To feel like every day has to be a study day can be so daunting for people that they get discouraged and give up. Such an approach is not necessary.

BIBLE READING

Daily Bible reading often has the following characteristics:

1. The primary goal is fellowship with God. This is your one-on-one time with the divine person who loves you more than you can imagine.

2. Find a translation that you enjoy and can relate to well. Over the years countless people have benefited from the *King James Version*, but many now stumble over the unfamiliar Elizabethan modes of expression. The *New King James Version* helps by updating the

language. Other translations like the *New International Version* take advantage of more recent archaeology and scholarship. Paraphrases, such as the Living Bible and The Message translate the text more loosely and are therefore not good choices for careful study, but can nonetheless be very beneficial for casual reading.

3. It is usually more helpful to focus on one book of the Bible at a time rather than randomly jumping around. Many people build a foundation with the Gospels and Acts first. After that, it can be useful to balance your time in the Old Testament and the New Testament. It is important to be familiar with all of Scripture, but portions of the Old Testament that contain long lists or intricate regulations such as Israel's ceremonial and civil laws probably won't fit the purpose of your reading time and are better reserved for study.

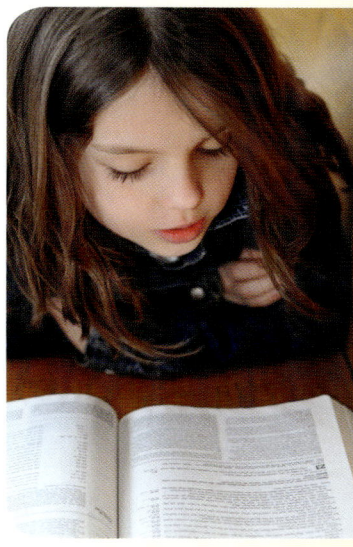

4. Take only a few verses at a time and let them soak into your soul. The goal is quality, not quantity. Just one verse can have a powerful impact. Whatever time you spend, divide it between reading and contemplation of the verses. Put yourself in any story as one of the characters and try to visualize the scene.

5. As you read, think about these questions.[52]

    a. What does the text tell me about God?

    b. What do these verses mean for me today? What area of my life can I trust God for more fully?

6. Keep a notebook handy to jot down your insights. Writing it down solidifies it in your mind. Also write down questions you may have of the text so you can go back and address them more in depth during your study time.

7. Memorize any verse that makes a particular impact on you and that you want to be able to refer back to mentally during the day.

BIBLE STUDY

Our focus now shifts from daily Bible reading to the more in-depth *study* you engage in at least once a week. How long you spend in each study session is not so much a matter of following a rigid schedule as it is taking enough time to gain new depths of understanding. You want to plunge significantly deeper than you normally would during a casual reading.

There are a number of ways to study Scripture. The following are some of the most common methods and approaches. It is important to vary your approach in order to keep yourself challenged and maintain interest.

All study methods mainly revolve around asking questions of the text. It can work well to use one or more of the standard questions – *Who? What? Where? When? How?* The more you ask, the more you will learn.[53]

Bible Study Method #1 – Bible Books
The key here is to keep your perspective on the overall theme of an entire book rather than examining individual chapters and verses. Read it through from beginning to end two or three times, continually asking, "Why was it written? What is the overarching purpose and theme?" You are looking for the big picture here.

Bible Study Method #2 – Bible Chapters and Verses
This strategy takes a book of the Bible and analyzes its parts, including the chapters and verses. Examine groups of verses that fall into natural segments. (Many Bibles will provide those groupings for you by inserting headings.) Study how the various segments in the book relate to each other and to other portions of Scripture. Look for key words and phrases. Think about original meanings and current applications.

Combine this approach with a study of the context within which the Bible teachings and events occurred. Take time to understand the history, geography, and culture of that period.

Bible Study Method #3 – Biographies
The focus is on one of the many fascinating people in Scripture. Locate the key verses pertaining to the individual. What were the major events in their life? What were the critical influences that shaped their attitudes and actions? What is it about them you want to emulate or avoid?

Bible Study Method #4 – Topics
Select a topic such as prayer, money, worship, truth, grace, law, redemption, etc., and follow it through Scripture.

Bible Study Method #5 – Character Traits
Choose a character trait such as faith, joy, patience, peace, love, endurance, hope, etc. What individuals exhibited these traits? In what circumstances do they show up? How are they developed?

Bible Study Tools
To get the most out of your study time, you will benefit from owning some of the following reference tools.

> *It can work well to use one or more of the standard questions — Who? What? Where? When? How? The more you ask, the more you will learn.*

BASIC TOOLS

1. **More than one translation of the Bible.** You may want to get a parallel Bible that has three or four versions side-by-side in one binding. Compare and contrast what each version says.

2. **Bible concordance.** This lists the words of Scripture alphabetically and the verses where they occur. Many Bibles have a concordance at the back, but they may not provide every occurrence of a word. To get that you will need what is called an *exhaustive* or *complete* concordance such as, Strong's or Cruden's. I would highly recommend the website: http://www.biblegateway.com for finding key words and verses in a variety of online translations. Also http://www.blueletterbible.org.

3. **Bible dictionary or encyclopedia.** These books explain many of the topics and practices of Bible times and also provide invaluable historical, geographic, and cultural background.[54] Three of the sources that I use are, *Encyclopedia of the Bible*, by Lion Publishing, *Everyday life in Bible Times*, by the National Geographic Society, and *Manners and Customs of Bible Times*, by Ralph Gower.

4. **A blank notebook.** It would be unfortunate to put in all this time and lose track of what you have learned. Keep notes of what impresses you the most. This journal will become an invaluable tool as you return to the same verses in the future.

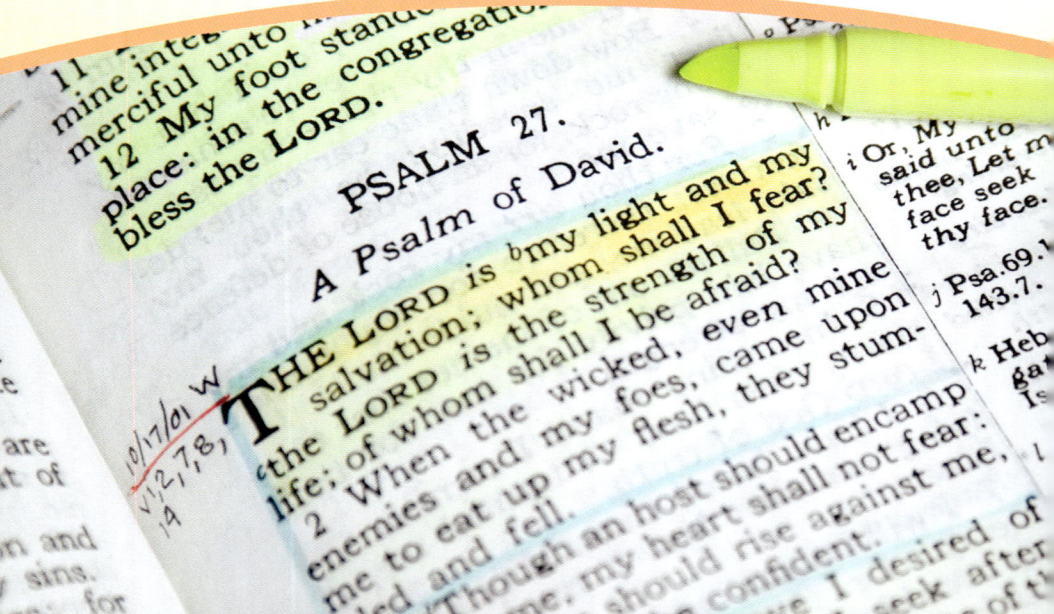

ADDITIONAL TOOLS

5. **Topical concordance.** Words of Scripture are grouped by topic.

6. **Harmony of the gospels.** Puts parallel verses from each gospel that cover the same incident or teaching side-by-side for easy comparison.

7. **Bible atlas.** Most Bibles have maps at the back, but an atlas will be much more exhaustive and have many more diagrams and illustrations. I personally enjoy the *Reader's Digest Atlas of the Bible*.

8. **Bible commentaries.** These are in-depth, verse by verse, studies of Scripture. It is preferable if each commentary you purchase covers only one book of the Bible. Some of my favorites are the commentaries that are part of the series entitled, "The New International Commentary on the New Testament."

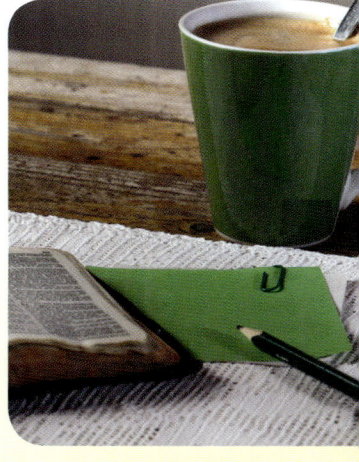

Jesus had an intimate knowledge of the Old Testament Scriptures. When he was twelve, he confounded Jewish leaders with his deep understanding. He also quoted Scripture repeatedly during his public ministry. It was his assimilation of Bible truth that lay at the foundation of his extraordinary trust in God. When that trust was severely tested at the beginning of his ministry, his defense was, "It is written . . ."

In the book of Acts, members of the church at Berea were commended because they "searched the scriptures daily, whether these things were so." As a result, "many of them believed" (see Acts 17:11–12, KJV).

We, too, can find an unshakable faith in God through a knowledge of the Bible. Like the savior and the Bereans, we can experience a deep, enduring trust that lifts us above the corrosive elements of this world and sustains us during difficult times. As Jesus promised, "You will know the truth, and the truth will set you free" (John 8:32, NIV).

DISCUSSION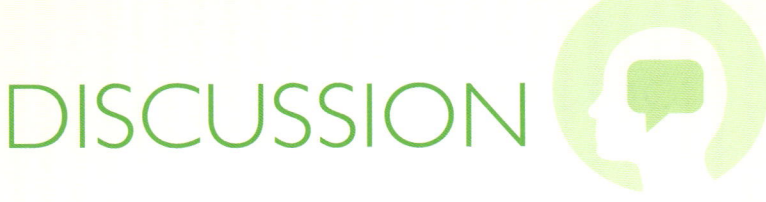

What has been a "roadblock" to Bible reading or study for you?
....
....

Has anyone ever taught you how to study the Bible? If so, what did they say?
....
....

What is your reaction to the difference between Bible reading and Bible study?
....
....

Share one of your favorite Bible verses or stories. Why is it so meaningful for you?
....
....

Describe a particularly impactful time you have had with Scripture lately.
....
....

What Bible verses would you use to help someone who felt discouraged?
....
....

Which of the five Bible study methods listed in the lesson do you find most appealing? How would you apply them to your own life?
....
....

What Bible study tools do you currently have? How do you use them? What tools might you consider adding?
....
....

SHARING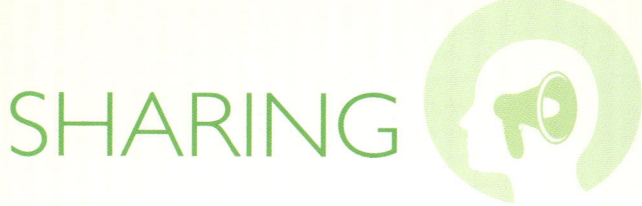

OPPORTUNITY #7:

- Pray as a group for God to open the way for you to share something from these lessons to help someone else.
- Keep your radar up each day for opportunities.

ABUNDANT LIVING THOUGHT

The Bible is the instruction manual on what trust in God is all about. It is the primary source.

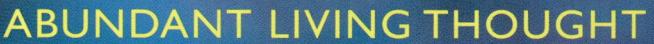

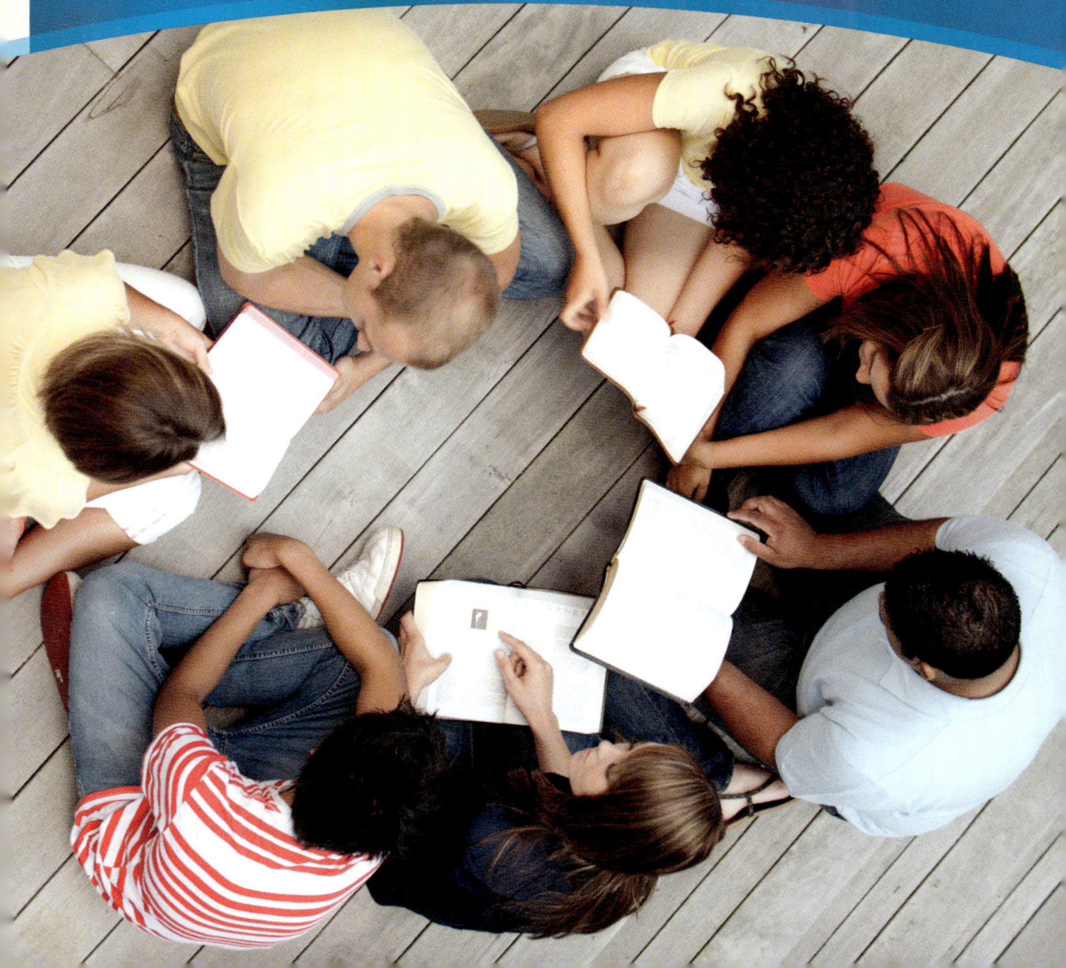

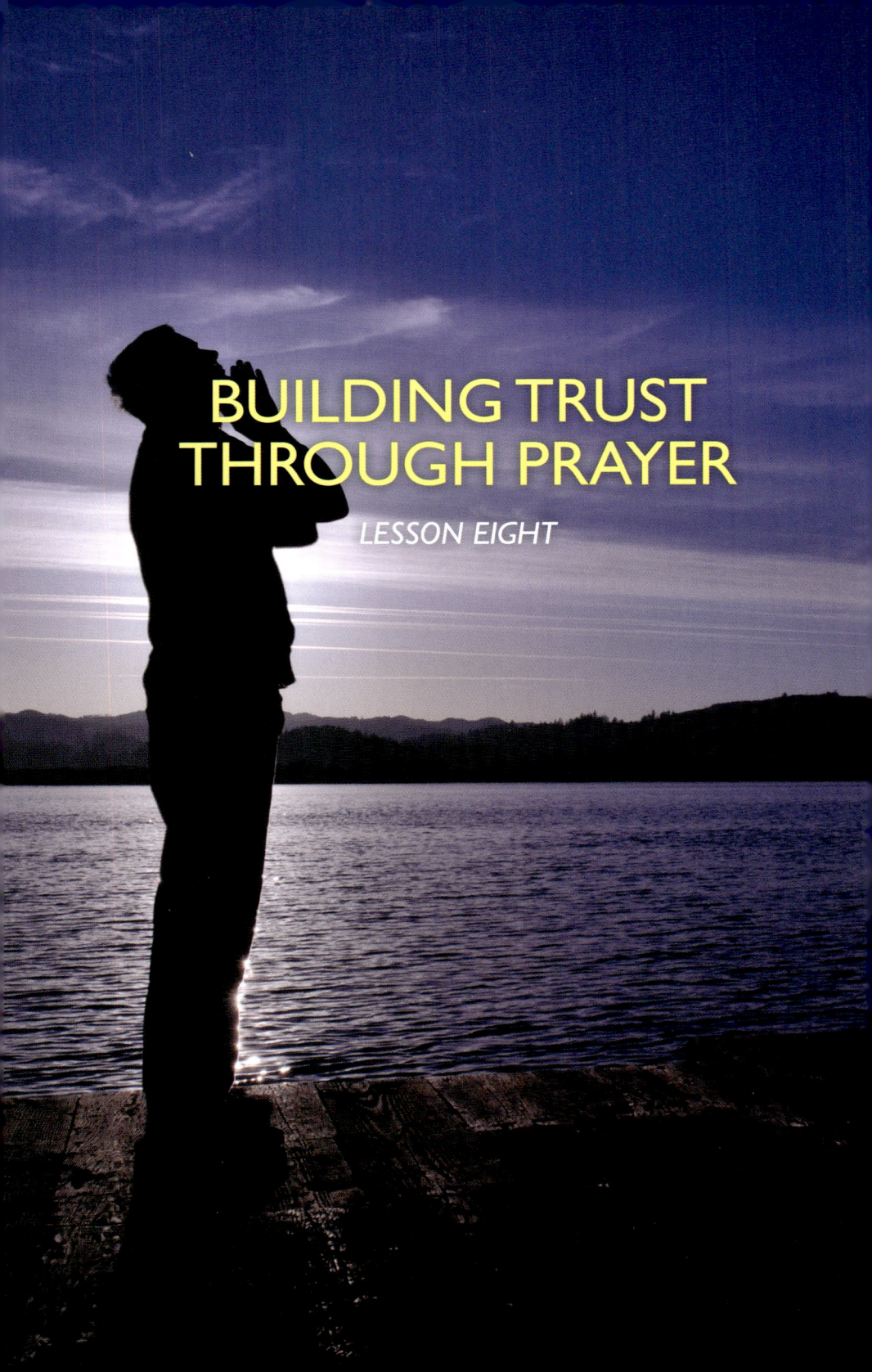

WARM UP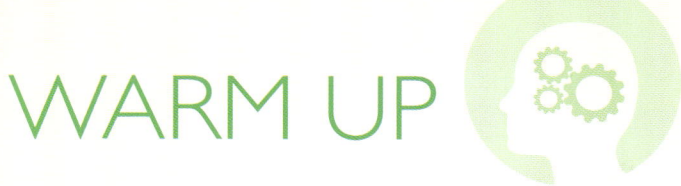

Feedback: In what ways did God open the door last week for you to share some part of the lessons with someone else?

....
....
....
....

Choose one or both questions to discuss (if in a group setting), or write out your answers on a separate sheet (for individual use):

1. **Share one of your most memorable moments as a member of this group.**

....
....
....

2. **What is one of the biggest things you have learned from these lessons? Why is that meaningful for you?**

....
....
....

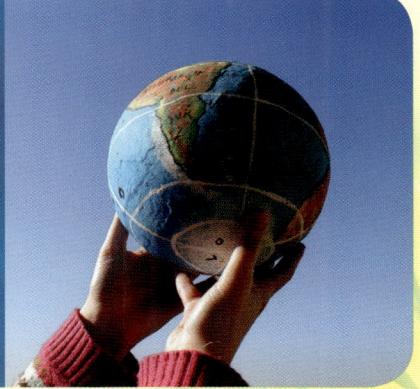

Very simply, prayer is relinquishing your greatest concerns to the Maker of the Universe.

MONICA REED, MD

DISCOVERY

I suddenly felt as if my world had been invaded by people with the very same weird affliction. First, there was the man at the supermarket pushing a half-filled cart down the cereal aisle who talked to himself loudly and with considerable urgency. He passed too quickly for me to catch more than, "I'll be late to the meeting at…" I stopped parallel to the granola section, turned, and did a long double take.

That same evening I visited the local mall to pick up some socks and passed by two more self-talkers. Over the next few days, I ran into several more at various venues. I had never before encountered such normal-looking individuals nonchalantly filling the air with solo verbiage.

"What on earth is going on?" I mused. Was there something in the water? Would I too be overcome with an uncontrollable urge to chat openly with a phantom partner? Finally, I overhead a tech-type person at work showing someone the new gadget he had purchased called a "Bluetooth." It was a tiny, hands free, cell phone accessory that hung on your ear like a hearing aid. They had gone on sale a short time before. *So that's what those people were up to*, I thought. I felt an immediate sense of amazement and relief. I was glad to know that there were actual people on the other end of those conversations.

To be honest, there are times when I feel like I am, in fact, talking to myself. That feeling comes periodically during my time in prayer.

I have heard others describe prayer as a "conversation" with God. What conversation? In all the time I've spent talking to God, I have never once heard him speak back to me audibly. I used to wonder if I was spiritually deficient. Was my religious receptor burned out? Were my prayers defective?

Through reading and experience, I have now developed a clearer idea of what prayer is and how it is intended to operate. *Over the years I have come to realize that, at its core, prayer is a vital pathway for building a trust relationship with God.* This lesson will explore some ways that can occur.

1. **Trusting that God hears.**

I now know that God listens when I pray and that I am not talking to myself even though it may seem that way. On many days I used to feel alone in prayer. But feelings are fickle and are not a reliable indicator.

I have confidence that God is present because of the many promises in Scripture that he hears us, like the one recorded by the psalmist David,

> *The righteous cry out, and the Lord hears,*
> *And delivers them out of all their troubles.*
> *The Lord is near to those who have a broken heart,*
> *And saves such as have a contrite spirit*
> *(Psalm 34:17–18, NKJV).*

Prayer is a great opportunity to build trust by leaning on God's promises instead of our own perceptions. Prayer enables us to exercise our trust muscles on a regular basis.

God is not "up there" somewhere. Our prayers do not "ascend" like some wireless text message to a distant friend. God is not limited by spatial considerations. He is right beside us, bending over us, with his ear inclined in our direction. Of course, he also hears just as clearly our thoughts and the unspoken yearnings of our heart.[55]

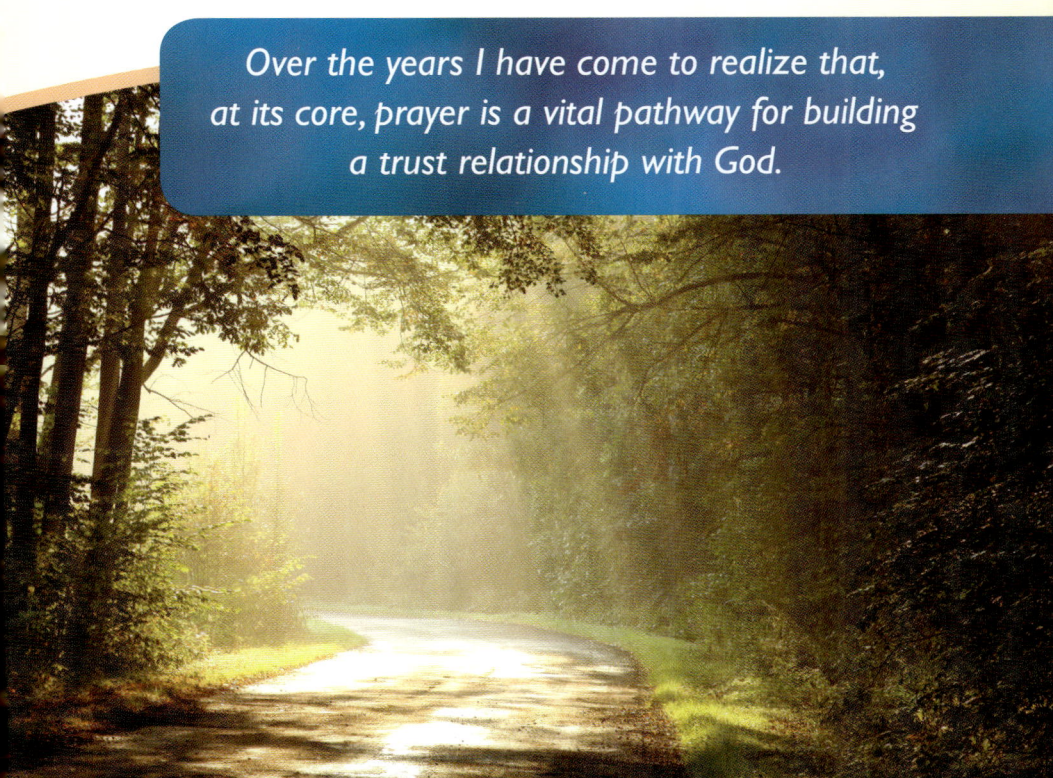

> *Over the years I have come to realize that, at its core, prayer is a vital pathway for building a trust relationship with God.*

2. Trusting that God does communicate.

I trust that God actually communicates with us based on what Jesus taught in the gospel of John, "When He, the Spirit of truth, has come, *He will guide you into all truth*" (John 16:13, NKJV, emphasis added). Rather than using an audible voice, his messages come to us more subtly through insights, impressions, and new understandings.

Prayer is probably when the Holy Spirit can speak to us best because he has our full attention. That is why prayer should be mostly about contemplation and listening rather than talking. God advises us through the psalmist, "Be still and know that I am God" (Psalm 46:10, NKJV). Mental stillness can be difficult to achieve because our world is not geared toward quietness. Instead it fills our brains with incessant talk and noise. Learning to quiet our minds is an art and skill that takes time and patience to accomplish, but the rewards are great.

That is also why prayer should be in a comfortable position physically. It is fine if getting on your knees to pray works best for you, but it is not essential. What is important is kneeling in our spirit to humbly pay attention. It can even be a good idea to have a notebook nearby.

> *We develop a deepening sense of confidence that he will indeed provide us with the insights and guidance we need as his followers.*

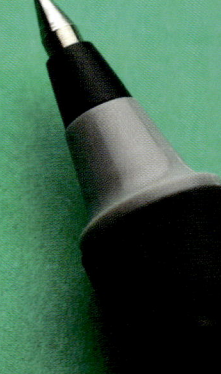

A set time for prayer is, of course, not the only time the Holy Spirit can communicate with us. He can teach us as we offer spontaneous mini-prayers and as we maintain a sense of God's presence throughout the day.

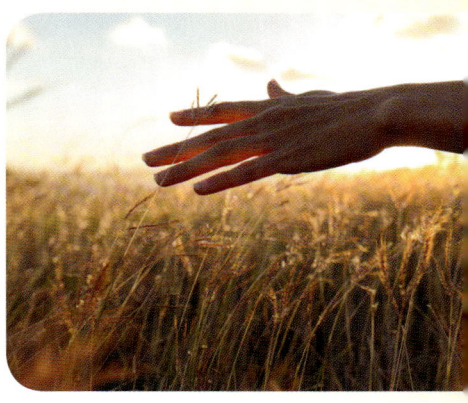

Over time our trust builds as we come to realize that God is, in fact, actively sharing with us. We develop a deepening sense of confidence that he will indeed provide us with the insights and guidance we need as his followers.

As much as I believe in the Spirit's willingness to communicate, I have to admit that I get a little nervous when people throw around the phrase "God told me" too glibly. Such a statement can be used to justify all kinds of bad decisions. So how can we distinguish the voice of the Spirit from the aberrant thoughts that come from simply eating too much pizza?

That is a large topic, but a few brief points may help. I think in terms of three categories:

> **Level #1 – Learning Scripture.** I trust that the Spirit is involved in any insights I gain about how to understand Scripture.
>
> **Level #2 – Applying Scripture.** I trust that the Spirit is the one who helps me understand how to apply Bible teachings to my life. He convicts me when changes are in order and reminds me of the promises of Scripture regarding forgiveness, salvation, and spiritual growth.
>
> **Level #3 – Life Decisions.** This final category is where things can get a little dicey, especially if others are affected. The more impactful our intention, the more we need to seek counsel from others and proceed only when we find a consensus. That is why God has provided the church, the Body of Christ, to give us guidance. The Holy Spirit works with us individually, but he also works through the wisdom of a community of believers as well. The Spirit also works through professionals to steer our course when appropriate.

3. Trusting God with our deepest secrets.

One of the surest ways to bond more deeply with a person is to trust them with a secret that you assiduously keep from others. Such sharing takes the relationship to a whole new level. It is a rare and special privilege to have someone manifest enough confidence in you to share so personally.

Sharing secrets is not only preceded by extraordinary trust in another individual, it also builds even greater trust. Sharing at such an intimate level expands the quality and dimensions of trust by allowing it to encompass more of who we are.

Most relationships never get beyond the relatively safe level of sharing ideas and opinions. Other times we may share more of ourselves with a smaller group by talking about our feelings. But secrets are usually limited to the closest one or two friends – a longtime ally or a spouse.

Even then, other secrets can remain that do not get shared at all. They need not be something illegal or morally wrong. They can simply be hurts or insecurities that we dare not share with anyone for fear of being rejected, ridiculed, or shamed.

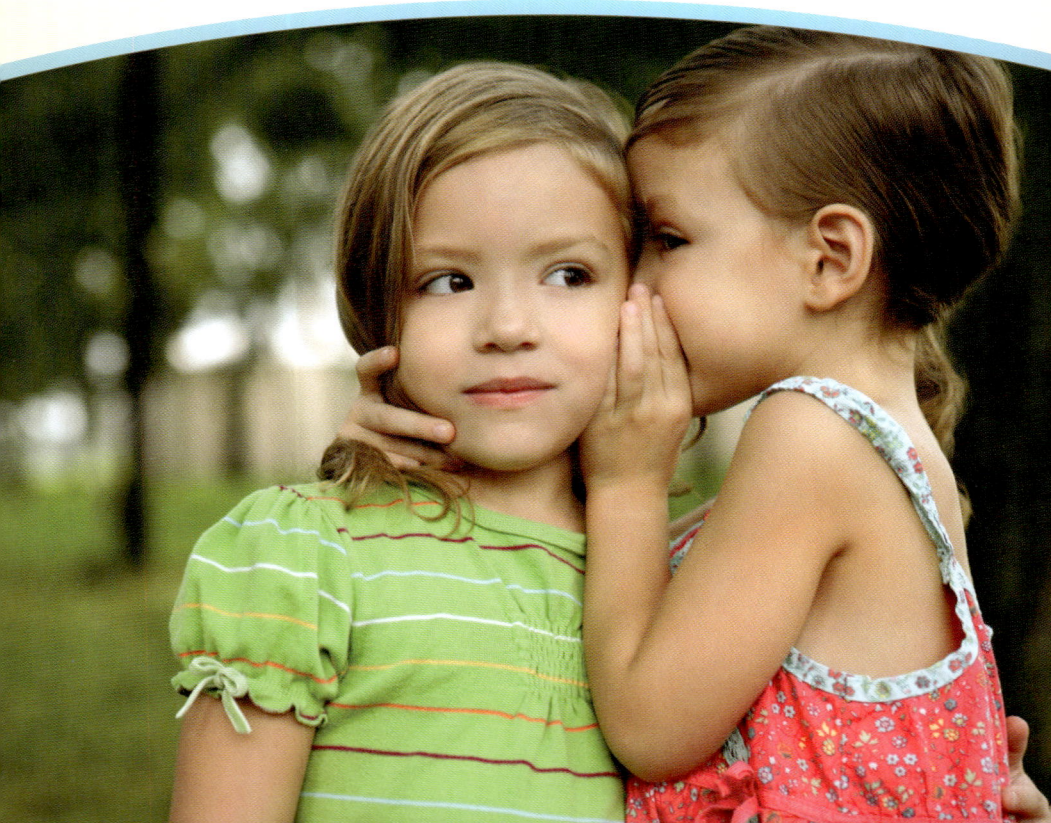

It is these very issues that we can always safely share with God. He is anxious to hear it all and will never react in a negative or condescending way. And as we share these deepest needs, our trust in God grows. Each time we tell him what we can tell no one else, we become more willing to trust him further.

Philip Yancey writes, "Prayer makes room for the unspeakable, those secret compartments of shame and regret that we seal away from the outside world … In truth, what I think and feel as I pray, rather than the words I speak, may be the real prayer … And as I learn to give voice to those secrets, mysteriously the power they hold over me melts away."[56]

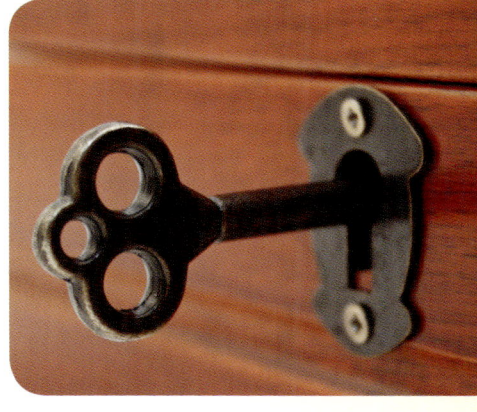

In the gospels, we read about a man named Nicodemus, a well-known Pharisee, who shared some secrets with the savior. He was so embarrassed that he came to Christ after dark in an out-of-the-way location. He may even have whispered his questions and concerns after nervously checking that they were, in fact, alone. This long-time religious leader felt he could confide in the young rabbi from Nazareth because he had witnessed Jesus' keen insight and great compassion. The savior sat still and listened with enormous empathy, never letting his gaze stray from the unsettled man before him.

That night of close sharing initiated what became an extraordinary level of trust within the heart of Nicodemus. He had such confidence in the savior that he later defended him before the Jewish authorities and then helped Joseph of Arimathea prepare Jesus' body for burial in Joseph's tomb. (see John 3:1–21; 7:50; 19:39).

> *As we share these deepest needs, our trust in God grows. Each time we tell him what we can tell no one else, we become more willing to trust him further.*

4. Trusting God enough to share our true feelings.

I was feeling increasingly frustrated with one of my closest friends. He is a very interesting, fun-loving guy. We have shared many in-depth discussions about a variety of topics and often laughed until our sides hurt.

But he had this annoying habit of talking over me and finishing my sentences. My frustration grew over time until one day I decided to let him know how I honestly felt. The next time he did it, I interrupted him and said, "Halt, time out. I've got something I need to share." I told him what was bothering me and concluded by saying, "Let me put it this way – here's a new rule. Whenever my lips are moving, yours aren't."

He seemed momentarily stunned. Then he leaned back and laughed like crazy. "I get it," he offered. "Sorry." I only see him infrequently now, but whenever I do, he always starts the conversation by saying, "Don't worry, when you're lips are moving, mine won't."

Close friends are able to share their true feelings. The greater the trust, the greater the willingness to say exactly how we feel, which in turn leads to even stronger trust.

The same holds true for our relationship with God. In prayer, instead of saying, "Lord, I am a little annoyed at you today," tell him, "I'm furious at you for what happened!" Instead of saying, "I feel a little down today," tell him, "I feel like giving up!" Get it out. He knows what we are going to tell him anyway. Jesus wants us to share for our sake, not his. And the more genuine our sharing, the more our trust in him will grow.[57]

One cannot read the Psalms without being impressed by the complete honesty of David, the author of many of them. His feelings run the gamut from joy to utter despair. He both praises God and denounces him. For example:

> *But to You I have cried out, O Lord,*
> *And in the morning my prayer comes before You.*
> *Lord, why do You cast off my soul?*
> *Why do You hide Your face from me?*
> *I have been afflicted and ready to die from my youth;*
> *I suffer Your terrors;*
> *I am distraught*
> *(Psalm 88:13–15, NKJV).*

Such openness was born of the very close connection David had with his redeemer.

God understands well the full range of human emotions. He knows that his followers are not immune from highs and lows. He delights in our good days and responds to our bad days with great empathy and grace.

5. Trusting that prayer changes us.

Prayer is not primarily about getting what we want. It is, rather, a special opportunity to put ourselves in a frame of mind and heart where God can reach down and change us.[58] That change happens through prayer in a variety of ways:

   a. The more we dwell on the character of God in prayer, the more we become like him (see 2 Cor. 3:18).

   b. Prayer permanently impacts our thought processes as we mentally spend time in God's alternative kingdom where his values and priorities take center stage.

   c. Prayer enables us to reframe life events and circumstances and view them from God's perspective.

   d. It gives us an opportunity to recalibrate our lives and make sure we are putting first things first.

These inner changes take time and are not immediately obvious, but trust tells us that they are nonetheless very real.

The following quote summarizes well the value of prayer, "I pray in astonished belief that God desires an ongoing relationship. I pray in trust that the act of prayer is God's designated way of closing the vast gulf between infinity and me. I pray in order to put myself in the stream of God's healing work on earth."[59]

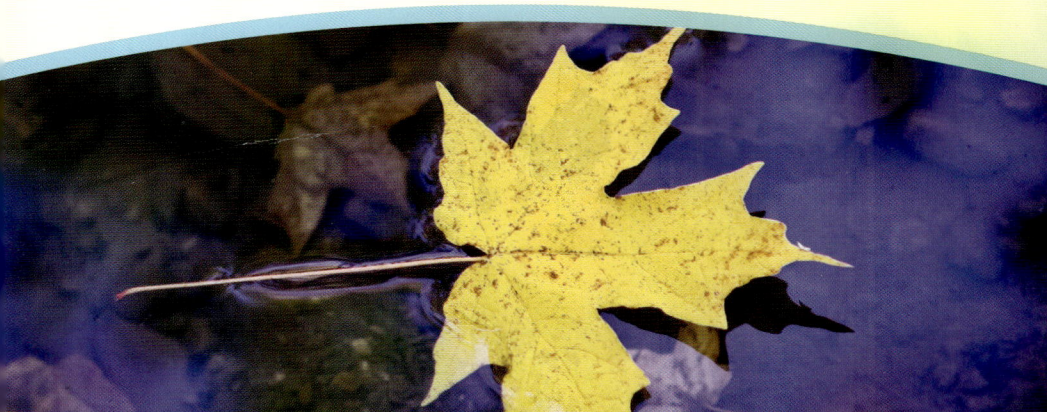

DISCUSSION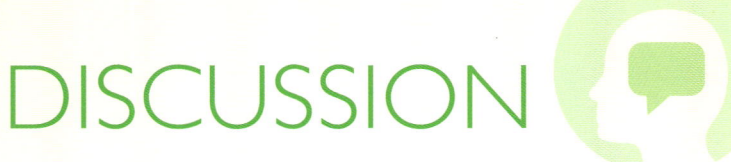

Do you ever feel like you are talking to yourself in prayer? What helps?
....
....

What are some different ways we can communicate with God?
....
....

Describe your mental picture of what God is doing when you pray.
....
....

Is prayer meaningful for you? Why or why not?
....
....

How confident are you that God communicates with you? Why?
....
....

What thoughts has God been impressing you with lately?
....
....

Are you comfortable telling God exactly how you feel? Why or why not?
....
....

What are some ways to keep prayer from becoming a dull routine?
....
....

SHARING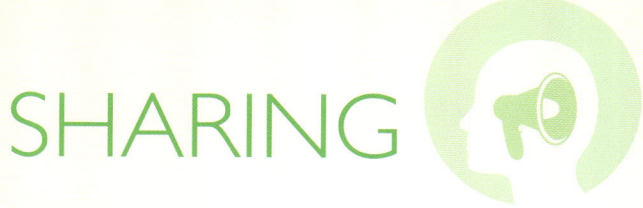

OPPORTUNITY #8:

- Pray as a group for God to open the way for you to share something from these lessons to help someone else.
- Keep your radar up each day for opportunities.

ABUNDANT LIVING THOUGHT

God delights in our good days and responds to our bad days with great empathy and grace.

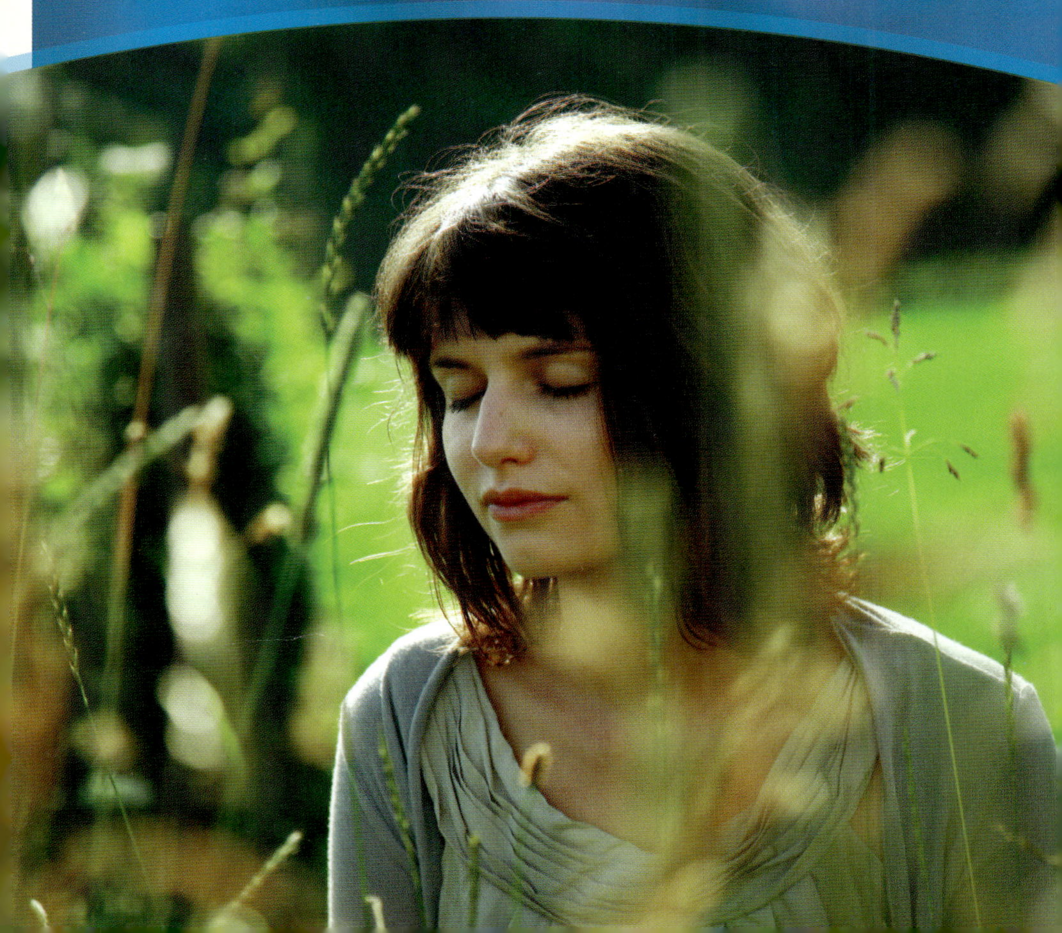

NOTES:

ABOUT THE AUTHOR

Kim Johnson is a popular writer, speaker, and fervent advocate for holistic living. As the author of three books, eleven lesson series, and many articles, his writings focus on healthy living and spiritual connectedness. His materials have been used in hundreds of churches throughout North America and internationally as well.

Johnson is an ordained minister with more than 35 years of experience as a parish pastor and church administrator. Over the years, his work with parishioners emphasized principles of whole-person health as a path to optimum mental, physical, social, and spiritual well-being. His later work with pastors and church leaders emphasized skill development such as vision casting, goal setting, support systems, relationship management, and accountability. Johnson has put his experience of working with pastors and parishioners to use in the CREATION Health Life Guide Series by creating a resource ideally suited for use in churches, small groups or individual study.

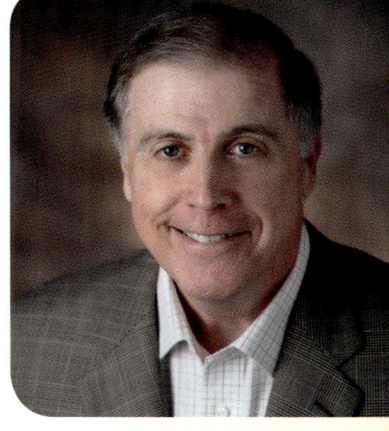

Johnson holds a Master of Divinity degree and received his Bachelor of Arts in theology. He currently serves as Director of Resource Development for churches in the state of Florida. His personal interests include reading, classical music, art and book festivals, kayaking, traveling, volunteering, and small group study. He and his wife Ann make their home in Orlando.

Author Acknowledgements: It has been a great privilege for me to be associated with the team of dedicated individuals who helped in various ways to make these CREATION Health Life Guides available. I would like to single out my wife Ann and daughter Stefanie, whose feedback and suggestions were always characterized by unfailing support and clear-eyed honesty. I have also received invaluable guidance and encouragement from Mike Cauley, Tim Nichols, Nick Howard, and Jim Epperson. Finally, I want to thank the group of local pastors who met with me personally and provided a wonderful forum for evaluating the lesson drafts.

NOTES

1. Garry Poole, *The Complete Book of Questions* (Grand Rapids, MI: Zondervan, 2003), 37.
2. Ibid., 41.
3. Ibid., 118.
4. Barbara Ann Kipfer, *4,000 Questions For Getting to Know Anyone and Everyone* (New York, NY: Random House Reference, 2004), 47.
5. John MacArthur, *Twelve Ordinary Men* (Nashville, TN: W. Publishing Group, 2002), 152.
6. Reader's Digest, *Jesus and His Times* (Pleasantville, NY: The Reader's Digest Association, 1987), 112.
7. Ibid., 112.
8. William Barclay, *The Gospel of Mark* (Philadelphia, PA: The Westminster Press, 1975), 302.
9. Norval Geldenhuys, *Commentary On the Gospel of Luke* (Grand Rapids, MI: Wm. B. Eerdmans Publishing Company, 1977), 520–521; William Barclay, *The Gospel of Luke* (Philadelphia, PA: The Westminster Press, 1975), 254–256.
10. Barclay, *Gospel of Mark*, 273–274.
11. William Barclay, *The Gospel of Matthew, Volume 2* (Philadelphia, PA: The Westminster Press, 1975), 247; William L. Lane, *The Gospel According to Mark* (Grand Rapids, MI: William B. Eerdmans Publishing Company, 1974), 406–407.
12. Kipfer, *4,000 Questions*, 124.
13. Brennan Manning, *Ruthless Trust* (New York, NY: Harper One, 2000), 97.
14. Frederick William Danker, *Greek-English Lexicon of the New Testament and Other Early Christian Literature* (Chicago, IL: The University of Chicago Press, 2000), 819.
15. "How Night Vision Works," Jeff Tyson, How Stuff Works, accessed November 12, 2012, http://electronics.howstuffworks.com/gadgets/high-tech-gadgets/nightvision.htm.
16. Kipfer, *4,000 Questions*, 61.
17. Leon Morris, *The Gospel According to Matthew* (Grand Rapids, MI: William B. Eerdmans Publishing Company, 1992), 188.
18. William Barclay, *The Gospel of Matthew, Volume One* (Louisville, KY: Westminster John Knox Press, 2001), 341.
19. Kipfer, *4,000 Questions*, 31.
20. Poole, *Complete Book of Questions*, 122.
21. Jeffrey S. Levin and Linda M. Chatters, "Religion, Health, and Psychological Well-Being in Older Adults: Findings from Three National Surveys," *Journal of Aging and Health* 10, no. 4 (Nov. 1998), 504–531.
22. Harold G. Koenig, *Medicine Religion and Health* (West Conshohocken, PA, Templeton Foundation Press, 2008), 78–79.
23. David B. Larson, Harold G. Koenig, Berton H. Kaplan, Raymond S. Greenberg, Everett Logue, and Herman A. Tyroler, "The Impact of Religion on Men's Blood Pressure," *Journal of Religion and Health* 28, no. 4 (Winter 1989), 263–278.

24. Jeff Levin, PhD, *God, Faith, and Health* (New York, NY: John Wiley & Sons, Inc., 2001), 132.
25. Ibid., 144.
26. Ellen L. Idler, "Religious Involvement and the Health of the Elderly: Some Hypotheses and an Initial Test," *Social Forces* 66 (1987), 226–238.
27. Levin, *God, Faith, and Health*, 137.
28. Monica Reed, MD, *The Creation Health Breakthrough* (New York, NY: Center Street, 2007), 124.
29. Des Cummings Jr., PhD, Monica Reed, MD, *Creation Health Discovery* (Maitland, FL: Florida Hospital Publishing, 2005), 65.
30. This concept comes from Corrie Ten Boom's poem, "The Weaving," found in her book, *The Hiding Place*, which was the basis of a 1975 film by the same name.
31. Michael Yaconelli, *Dangerous Wonder* (Colorado Springs, CO: NavPress, 2003), 64–66.
32. Poole, *Complete Book of Questions*, 93.
33. "What Are the Dead Sea Scrolls and Why Are They Important?" Got Questions?org, accessed November 12, 2012, http://www.gotquestions.org/dead-sea-scrolls.html.
34. Josh McDowell, *The New Evidence That Demands A Verdict* (Nashville, TN: Thomas Nelson Publishers, 1999), 78.
35. "Israel's War of Independence (1947–1949)," Israeli Ministry of Foreign Affairs, accessed November 12, 2012, http://www.mfa.gov.il/MFA/History/Modern+History/Israel+wars/Israels+War+of+Independence+-+1947+-+1949.htm.
36. "What Is the Importance of the Dead Sea Scrolls?" Dr. Will Varner, Christian Answers.net, accessed November 12, 2012, http://www.christiananswers.net/q-abr/abr-a023.html; Jeffery L. Sheler, *Is The Bible True?* (New York, NY: HarperCollins Publishers, Iinc., 1999), 128.
37. Erwin W. Lutzer, *Seven Reasons Why You Can Trust the Bible* (Chicago, IL: Moody Press, 1998), 83.
38. Jason Dulle, "Biblical Archaeology 32: The Dead Sea Scrolls," September 9, 2011, http://theosophical.wordpress.com/2011/09/09/biblical-archaeology-32-the-dead-sea-scrolls/.
39. "Formation of the Old Testament," Bread of Life Ministry, accessed November 12, 2012, http://breadoflifeministry.info/24422/86812.html.
40. "What Is the Importance of the Dead Sea Scrolls?" Varner, http://www.christiananswers.net/q-abr/abr-a023.html.
41. Gerhard Pfandl, PhD, "Is the Bible Historically Reliable," *Ministry* (Sept 2012), 23.
42. Del Ray Bible Institute, "Scripture and Hermeneutics," http://s3.amazonaws.com/churchplantmedia-cms/delreychurchca/drbi-hermeneutics-appendix-1.pdf.
43. Dr. John Ankerberg, Dr. John Welden, "The Historical Reliability of Scripture," http://www.ankerberg.com/Articles/editors-choice/EC1205W1.htm.
44. Abraham Smith, "The Birth of Christ: History or Myth?" http://lavistachurchofchrist.org/LVarticles/BirthOfChristFactOrMyth.html.
45. Josh McDowell, *The New Evidence That Demands A Verdict,* 93.

46. Sheler, *Is The Bible True?*, 59–60.
47. "Is the Bible Historically Accurate?" Daniel R. Vess, accessed November 13, 2012, http://www.forumterrace.com/Questions/Historically.html.
48. Sheler, *Is The Bible True?*, 112–113.
49. "Jesus Christ's Arrest, Trial and Crucifixion," Mario Seiglie, United Church of God, accessed November 13, 2012, http://www.churchofgodtwincities.org/lit/gn/gn028/trialcru.html; "Pontius Pilate Inscription," Great Archaeology, accessed November 13, 2012, http://www.greatarchaeology.com/Pontius.php.
50. Poole, *Complete Book of Questions*, 47.
51. Rick Warren, *Rick Warren's Bible Study Methods* (Grand Rapids, MI: Zondervan, 2006), 19.
52. Kay Arthur, David Arthur, Pete De Lacy, *The New How to Study Your Bible* (Eugene, OR: Harvest House Publishers, 2010), 11–13.
53. Ibid., 29–30.
54. "Bible Study Tools: Bible Dictionaries," Henry E. Neufeld, Energion, accessed November 13, 2012, http://books.energion.com/biblical/bible_dictionary.shtml.
55. "Can God Hear My Prayer?" Linda Gilden, CBN.com, accessed November 13, 2012, http://www.cbn.com/spirituallife/churchandministry/evangelism/Gilden_prayer.aspx.
56. Philip Yancey, *Prayer* (Grand Rapids, MI: Zondervan, 2006), 41.
57. "Honesty In Prayer," Mike Balog, SermonIndex.net, accessed November 13, 2012, http://www.sermonindex.net/modules/newbb/viewtopic.php?topic_id=12577&forum=34&3.
58. "Intercessory Prayer Changes Us, Not God," Dr. Gene Norris, *The Augusta Chronicle,* July 2, 2010, http://chronicle.augusta.com/life/your-faith/2010-07-02/intercessory-prayer-changes-us-not-god.
59. Yancey, *Prayer*, 326–327.

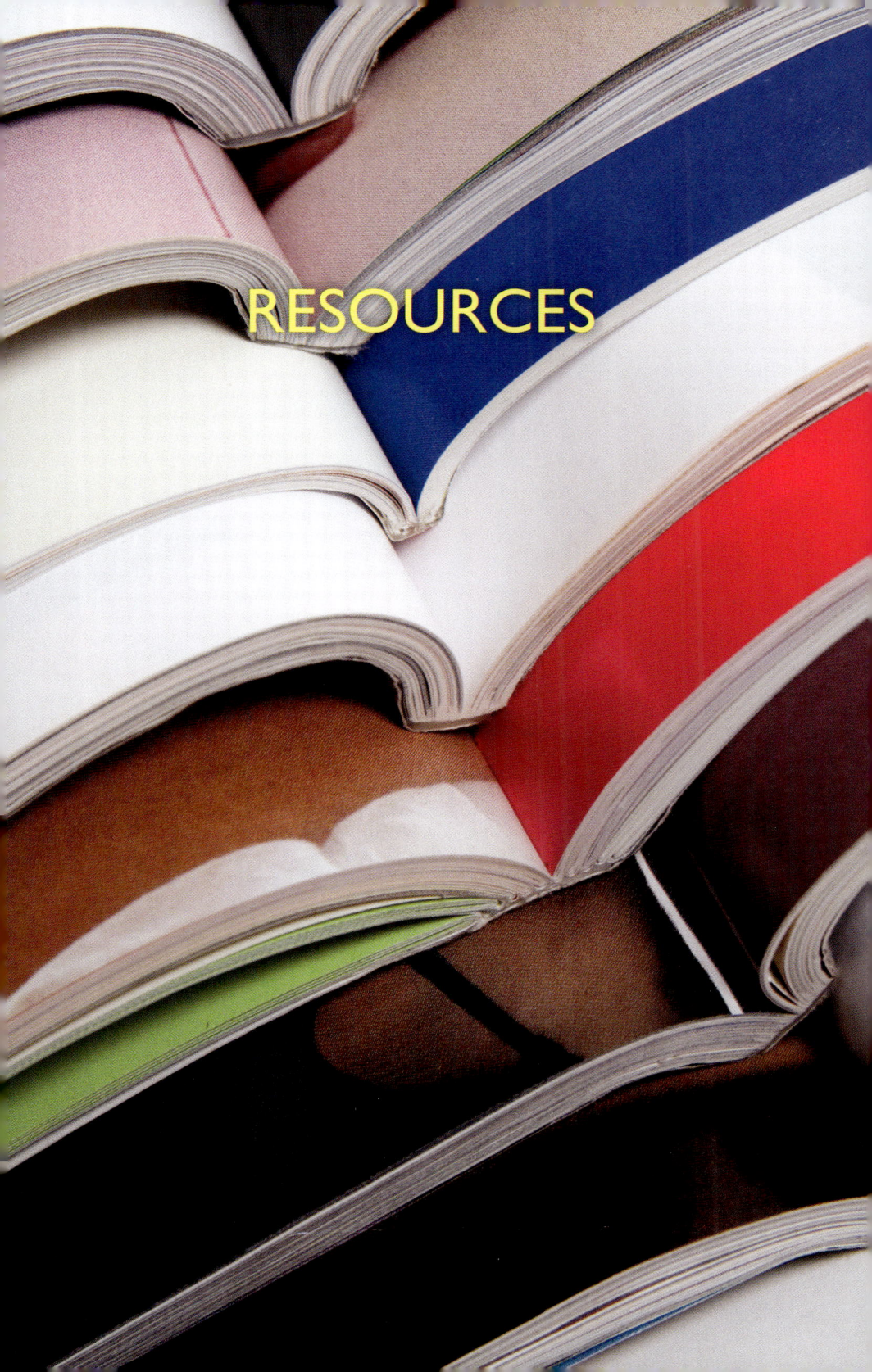

LEAD YOUR COMMUNITY
TO HEALTHY LIVING

CREATIONHealth.com — Shop online for CREATION Health Seminars, Books, & Resources

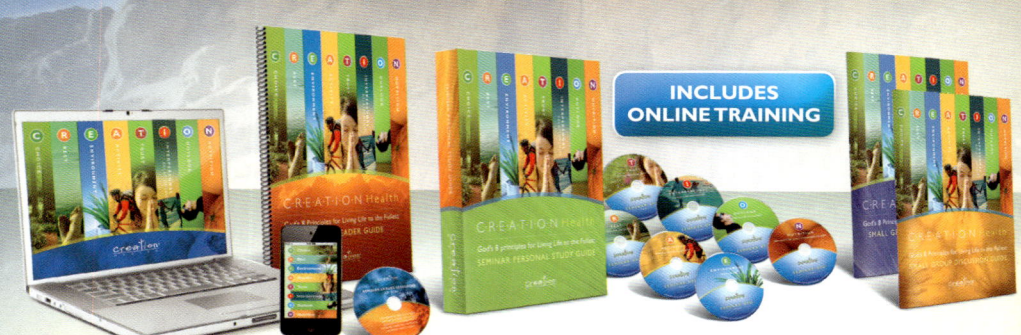

Seminar Leader Kit
Everything a leader needs to conduct this seminar successfully, including key questions to facilitate group discussion and PowerPoint presentations for each of the eight principles.

Participant Guide
A study guide with essential information from each of the eight lessons along with outlines, self assessments, and questions for people to fill-in as they follow along.

Small Group Kit
It's easy to lead a small group using the CREATION Health videos, the Small Group Leaders Guide and the Small Group Discussion Guide.

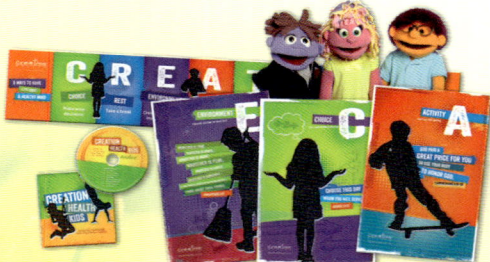

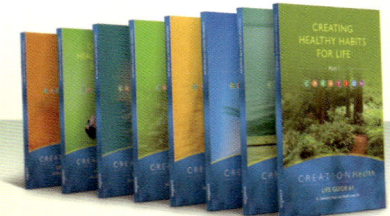

CREATION Kids
CREATION Health Kids can make a big difference in homes, schools and congregations. Lead kids in your community to healthier, happier living.

Life Guide Series
These guides include questions designed to help individuals or small groups study the depths of every principle and learn strategies for integrating them into everyday life.

GUIDES AND ASSESSMENTS

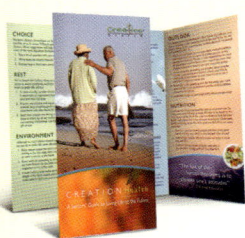
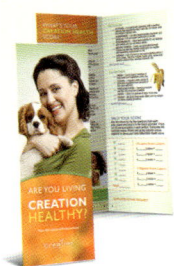
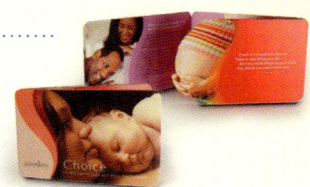

Pregnancy Guides
Expert advice on how to be CREATION Healthy while expecting.

Senior Guide
Share the CREATION Health principles with seniors and help them be healthier and happier as they live life to the fullest.

Self-Assessment
This instrument raises awareness about how CREATION Healthy a person is in each of the eight major areas of wellness.

Pocket Guide
A tool for keeping people committed to living all of the CREATION Health principles daily.

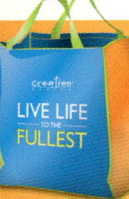

Tote Bag
A convenient way for bringing CREATION Health materials to and from class.

Tumbler
Practice good Nutrition and keep yourself hydrated with a CREATION Health tumbler in an assortment of fun colors.

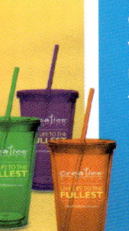

MARKETING MATERIALS

Postcards, Posters, Stationary, and more
You can effectively advertise and generate community excitement about your CREATION Health seminar with a wide range of available marketing materials such as enticing postcards, flyers, posters, and more.

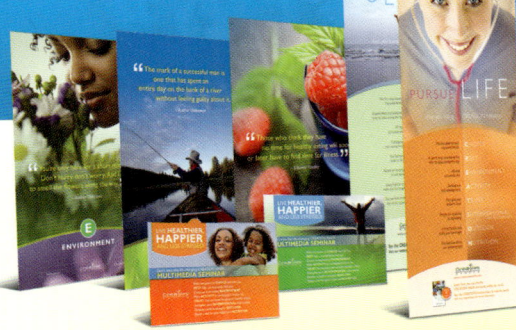

Bible Stories
God is interested in our physical, mental and spiritual well being. Throughout the Bible you can discover the eight principles for full life.

CREATION HEALTH BOOKS

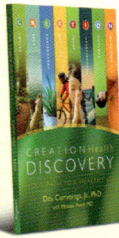

CREATION Health Discovery
Written by Des Cummings, Jr., PhD and Monica Reed, MD, this wonderful companion resource introduces people to the CREATION Health philosophy and lifestyle.

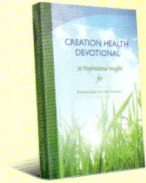

CREATION Health Devotional
In this devotional you will discover stories about experiencing God's grace in the tough times, God's delight in triumphant times, and God's presence in peaceful times.

English: Hardcover
Spanish: Softcover

CREATION HEALTH RESOURCES

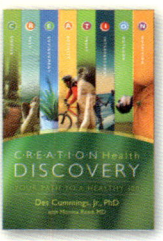

CREATION Health Discovery (Softcover)
CREATION Health Discovery takes the 8 essential principles of CREATION Health and melds them together to form the blueprint for the health we yearn for and the life we are intended to live.

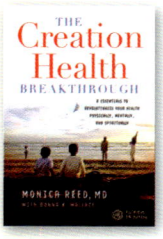

CREATION Health Breakthrough (Hardcover)
Blending science and lifestyle recommendations, Monica Reed, MD, prescribes eight essentials that will help reverse harmful health habits and prevent disease. Discover how intentional choices, rest, environment, activity, trust, relationships, outlook, and nutrition can put a person on the road to wellness. Features a three-day total body rejuvenation therapy and four-phase life transformation plan.

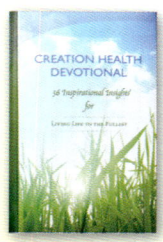

CREATION Health Devotional (English: Hardcover / Spanish: Softcover)
Stories change lives. Stories can inspire health and healing. In this devotional you will discover stories about experiencing God's grace in the tough times, God's delight in triumphant times, and God's presence in peaceful times. Based on the eight timeless principles of wellness: Choice, Rest, Environment, Activity, Trust, Interpersonal relationships, Outlook, Nutrition.

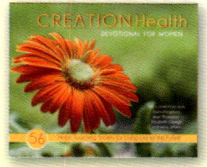

CREATION Health Devotional for Women (English)
Written for women by women, the *CREATION Health Devotional for Women* is based on the principles of whole-person wellness represented in CREATION Health. Spirits will be lifted and lives rejuvenated by the message of each unique chapter. This book is ideal for women's prayer groups, to give as a gift, or just to buy for your own edification and encouragement.

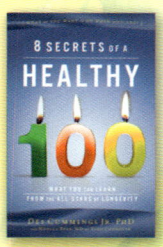

8 Secrets of a Healthy 100 (Softcover)
Can you imagine living to a Healthy 100 years of age? Dr. Des Cummings Jr., explores the principles practiced by the All-stars of Longevity to live longer and more abundantly. Take a journey through the 8 Secrets and you will be inspired to imagine living to a Healthy 100.

CREATION HEALTH RESOURCES

Forgive To Live (English: Hardcover / Spanish: Softcover)

In *Forgive to Live* Dr. Tibbits presents the scientifically proven steps for forgiveness – taken from the first clinical study of its kind conducted by Stanford University and Florida Hospital.

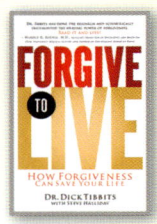

Forgive To Live Workbook (Softcover)

This interactive guide will show you how to forgive – insight by insight, step by step – in a workable plan that can effectively reduce your anger, improve your health, and put you in charge of your life again, no matter how deep your hurts.

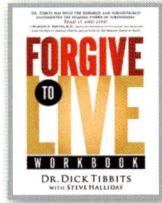

Forgive To Live Devotional (Hardcover)

In his powerful new devotional Dr. Dick Tibbits reveals the secret to forgiveness. This compassionate devotional is a stirring look at the true meaning of forgiveness. Each of the 56 spiritual insights includes motivational Scripture, an inspirational prayer, and two thought-provoking questions. The insights are designed to encourage your journey as you begin to *Forgive to Live*.

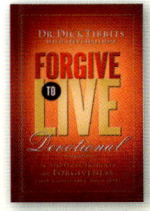

Forgive To Live God's Way (Softcover)

Forgiveness is so important that our very lives depend on it. Churches teach us that we should forgive, but how do you actually learn to forgive? In this spiritual workbook noted author, psychologist, and ordained minister Dr. Dick Tibbits takes you step-by-step through an eight-week forgiveness format that is easy to understand and follow.

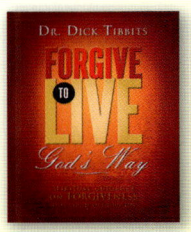

Forgive To Live Leader's Guide

Perfect for your community, church, small group or other settings.
The Forgive to Live Leader's Guide Includes:

- 8 Weeks of pre-designed PowerPoint™ presentations.
- Professionally designed customizable marketing materials and group handouts on CD-Rom.
- Training directly from author of Forgive to Live Dr. Dick Tibbits across 6 audio CDs.
- Media coverage DVD.
- CD-Rom containing all files in digital format for easy home or professional printing.
- A copy of the first study of its kind conducted by Stanford University and Florida Hospital showing a link between decreased blood pressure and forgiveness.

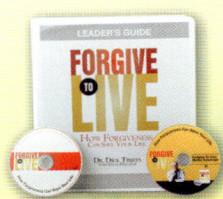

CREATION HEALTH RESOURCES

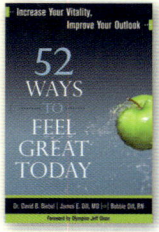

52 Ways to Feel Great Today (Softcover)

Wouldn't you love to feel great today? Changing your outlook and injecting energy into your day often begins with small steps. In *52 Ways to Feel Great Today*, you'll discover an abundance of simple, inexpensive, fun things you can do to make a big difference in how you feel today and every day. Tight on time? No problem. Each chapter is written as a short, easy-to-implement idea. Every idea is supported by at least one true story showing how helpful implementing the idea has proven to someone a lot like you. The stories are also included to encourage you to be as inventive, imaginative, playful, creative, or adventuresome as you can.

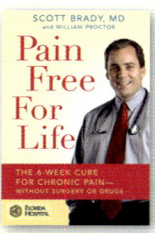

Pain Free For Life (Hardcover)

In *Pain Free For Life*, Scott C. Brady, MD, – founder of Florida Hospital's Brady Institute for Health – shares for the first time with the general public his dramatically successful solution for chronic back pain, Fibromyalgia, chronic headaches, Irritable bowel syndrome and other "impossible to cure" pains. Dr. Brady leads pain-racked readers to a pain-free life using powerful mind-body-spirit strategies used at the Brady Institute – where more than 80 percent of his chronic-pain patients have achieved 80-100 percent pain relief within weeks.

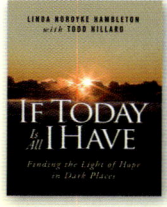

If Today Is All I Have (Softcover)

At its heart, Linda's captivating account chronicles the struggle to reconcile her three dreams of experiencing life as a "normal woman" with the tough realities of her medical condition. Her journey is punctuated with insights that are at times humorous, painful, provocative, and life-affirming.

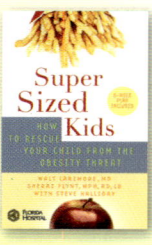

SuperSized Kids (Hardcover)

In *SuperSized Kids*, Walt Larimore, MD, and Sherri Flynt, MPH, RD, LD, show how the mushrooming childhood obesity epidemic is destroying children's lives, draining family resources, and pushing America dangerously close to a total healthcare collapse – while also explaining, step by step, how parents can work to avert the coming crisis by taking control of the weight challenges facing every member of their family.

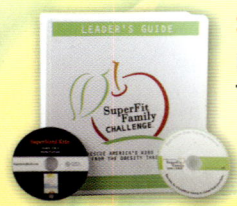

SuperFit Family Challenge – Leader's Guide

Perfect for your community, church, small group or other settings.
The SuperFit Family Challenge Leader's Guide Includes:
- 8 Weeks of pre-designed PowerPoint™ presentations.
- Professionally designed marketing materials and group handouts from direct mailers to reading guides.
- Training directly from Author Sherri Flynt, MPH, RD, LD, across 6 audio CDs.
- Media coverage and FAQ on DVD.

LIVE YOUR LIFE TO THE FULLEST

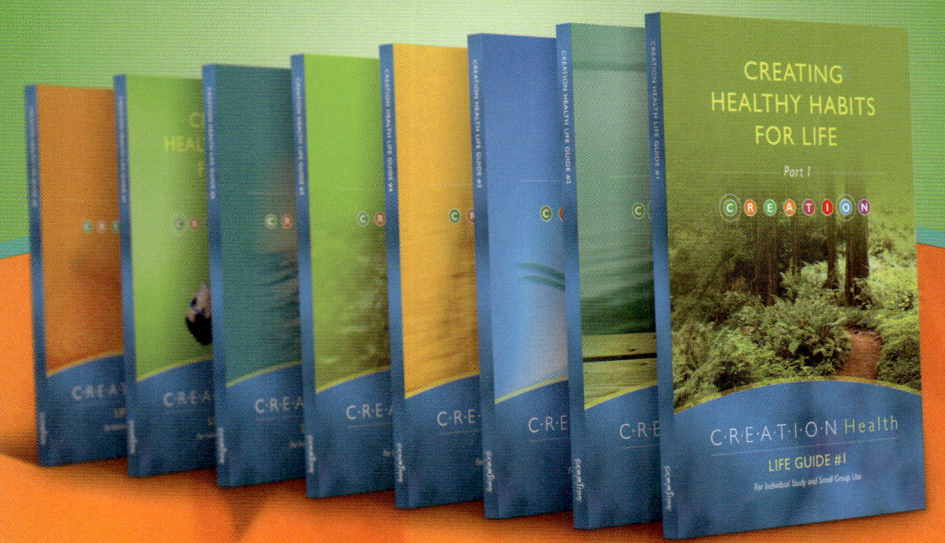

C·R·E·A·T·I·O·N Health

LIFE GUIDE SERIES

8 Guides. 8 Principles. One Powerful Message.
Packed with fresh insights on abundant living.
For Individual Study and Small Group Use.

Perfect for churches, schools, universities, and faith-based businesses.

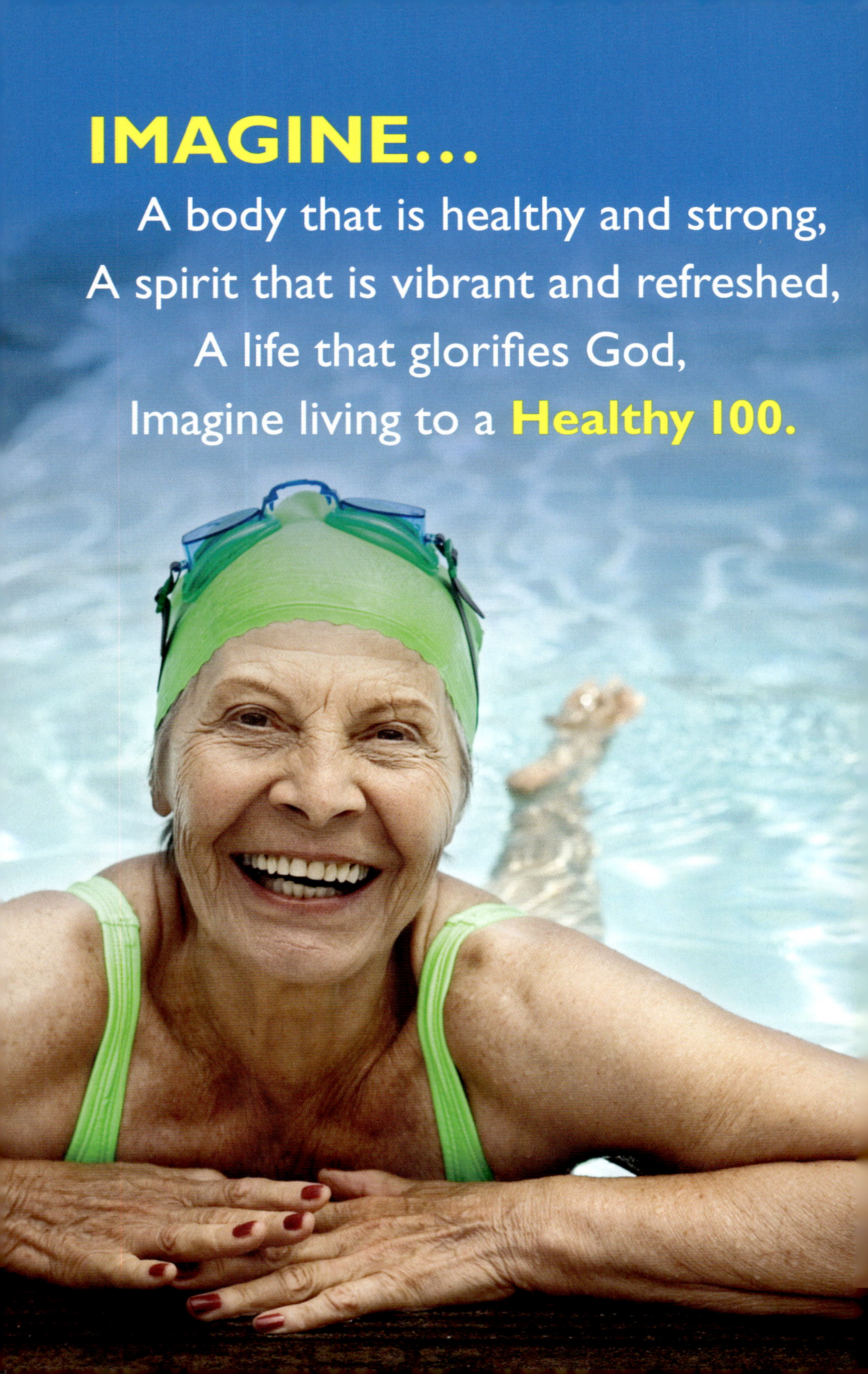

IMAGINE…

A body that is healthy and strong,
A spirit that is vibrant and refreshed,
A life that glorifies God,
Imagine living to a **Healthy 100**.

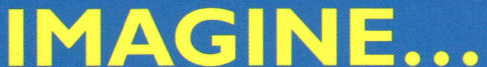